D0035398

Suicide by Sugar

A Startling Look at Our #1 National Addiction

Nancy Appleton, PhD

G.N. Jacobs

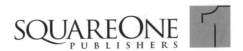

SQUAREONE
PUBLISHERS

COVER DESIGNER: Jeannie Tudor
EDITOR: Michele D'Altorio
TYPESETTER: Gary A. Rosenberg

The information and advice contained in this book are based upon the research and the personal and professional experiences of the authors. They are not intended as a substitute for consulting with a healthcare professional. The publisher and author are not responsible for any adverse effects or consequences resulting from the use of any of the suggestions, preparations, or procedures discussed in this book. All matters pertaining to your physical health should be supervised by a healthcare professional. It is a sign of wisdom, not cowardice, to seek a second or third opinion.

Square One Publishers
115 Herricks Road • Garden City Park, NY 11040
(516) 535-2010 • (877) 900-BOOK • www.squareonepublishers.com

Credit Line:
Cartoons on pages 20, 28, and 106 have been reprinted with permission from CSL, CartoonStock Ltd.

Library of Congress Cataloging-in-Publication Data
Appleton, Nancy.
  Suicide by sugar : a startling look at our #1 national addiction / Nancy Appleton, G.N. Jacobs.
     p. cm.
  Includes bibliographical references and index.
  ISBN 978-0-7570-0306-6
  1. Sugar–Pathophysiology. 2. Homeostasis. 3. Nutritionally induced diseases. 4. Food allergy. 5. Food–Sugar content. I. Jacobs, G. N. II. Title.
  RC627.R43A674 2009
  616.3'998–dc22

                              2009007800

Printed in the United States of America

10   9   8   7   6   5   4

Contents

Other Titles by Nancy Appleton

The Curse of Louis Pasteur

Healthy Bones

Lick the Sugar Habit

Lick the Sugar Habit Sugar Counter

Stopping Inflammation (with G.N. Jacobs)

*This book is dedicated to all
the people who have not found answers
to their health problems.*

*And also, to my children Laurie and Greg,
who have loved me and accepted, supported,
and followed my health ideas.
They have been blessings in my life.*

- N.A.-

Introduction

Y ou are about to venture on a journey about sugar, its effects on your body, and what you can do to change your habits. Some of the information you'll pick up along this journey will shock you, other information will enlighten you, but above all, you will finish the journey knowing exactly what you can do to avoid committing suicide by sugar.

Before you begin your journey, you should know that today, when people say "sugar" or "sucrose," they are usually referring to the sweetener made by beet, cane, and corn. The sugar and corn sweetener industries, however, do not do this. To the industries, "sugar" comes from beet or cane, not corn. "Sweetener" or "corn sweetener," to the industries, means it comes from corn. In this book, I use the word "sugar" to mean the substance that comes from beet, cane, and corn, except in the section titled "Fructose Roulette" (see page 60), where I speak specifically about sugar (beet or cane) and corn sweetener.

Your journey begins with my story. As a sugar addict, I came close to committing sugar suicide. I would quit but then go back to sugar, and you probably will also. Don't blame yourself. Just say, "Tomorrow will be a better day," and it will. Many of you will identify with my story. Over the years, I have heard variations of my story from many people.

The core of my early work started from the proposition that many people who eat too much sugar are sick too much of the time. I certainly was. After many years of abusing my body with sugar (unknowingly), I finally came to the conclusion that sugar must do something bad to the immune system. I researched a concept called homeostasis (the balance of all the systems in the body), and bingo, the whole story came together. I found out that sugar upsets this delicate balance in the body. I also learned what sugar does to the immune system.

The next stop along your journey will take you into new territory. First, you will learn all the ways sugar is ruining your health. Next, I will tell you exactly what I discovered about sugar's effect on homeostasis and the immune system. Then, you will find out about the glycemic index, glycemic load, and the importance of not taking an oral glucose tolerance test. You will also learn about Ensure and Pediasure, and you'll find out some information about soft drinks that you may not want to know. Additionally, you will discover how much natural sugar is in many products and how much sugar is added. There are also a few misconceptions about chocolate that are documented.

Next, I explain that sugar and its cousins (like honey, maple syrup, corn syrup, fructose, glucose, and others) can lead to a host of diseases. You will learn how sugar feeds cancer, dementia, and epilepsy, to name a few. Hypoglycemia (low blood sugar) is explained in depth.

After you discover what sugar does to the body, you will find out how to remove this sugar and keep it out of your body. There is a whole section on helping you get and stay healthy with food plans, suggestions for snacks, and recipes to soothe the sweet tooth. And there is more—much more.

Research into sugar has exploded in recent years, and it's not just crank nutritionists, dentists, and chemists doing the work—a few MDs are getting into the act as well. This represents a titanic shift in medical opinion, at least for the average doctor on the street. Even though the American Medical Association (AMA) has not directly come out against sugar, some of the associations for the many specialties contained within the AMA have made statements about sugar. Clearly, it is a case of waiting for the dinosaurs to die off.

So read on, dear reader, to start your journey and find out information that you did not know existed about sugar. If by the end of this book you haven't decided to lick your sugar habit, illness and a long, slow death may result—truly *Suicide by Sugar*.

1

Confessions of a Sugarholic

Hello. My name is Nancy Appleton and I am a recovering sugarholic.

I decided to drastically eliminate sugar from my diet to save my life in the 1970s after suffering from bad health and frequent illnesses for years. No other remedies were working, and since I had heard that many people who eat too much sugar are sick too much of the time, it seemed like the logical thing to do. My experiment with my health began because nothing ever got better until I worked on my sugar intake. As I started to feel better than I ever had before in my life, I ran into a wall of ignorance and willful blindness that still afflicts some areas of the medical and nutrition fields.

The notion that eating sugar in large quantities has a negative impact on one's health isn't one that is widely recognized and accepted. Then again, there are plenty of things that people used to know nothing about. For example, smoking has only officially been bad for you since the 1990s. Three-point safety harnesses for cars have only been standard equipment for about the same amount of time. And helmet requirements for motorcycles and bicycles? Forget about it. I hope that sometime soon eating sugar in large quantities will also be looked upon as ancient history.

This section of the book documents my journey through life as a sugar addict and explains why I made the decision to eliminate sugar from my diet.

ADDICTED FROM AN EARLY AGE

Before I knew why I was sick, I was an addict. A sugarholic, if you need a label for it.

I have vivid memories of the bakery truck that rumbled by the back door of my childhood house. I would charge donuts, nut bars, and coffee cakes to the household account. I hid the booty and let my mom deal with the bill, which was never itemized in enough detail for me to get caught. Does this sound like addictive behavior? Well, we call it alcoholism when a future AA member hides beer around the house. Anyway, the bakery goods were gone in two days and I would eagerly await the truck's return.

From those early years on, disease stalked me. I kept my doctors busy. I suffered my first bout of pneumonia at thirteen, and seemed to get relapses on an average of once every few years. Boils, canker sores, varicose veins, headaches, yeast infections, fatigue, colds, allergies, and influenza all led to six more pneumonia spells before I turned forty.

In my second year of college, doctors yanked a tumor out of my chest that was composed of pure calcium. I still couldn't make the connection that the amount of sugar I was consuming was seriously affecting my body. I was confused—since my early teens I was busy playing tennis for four hours a day, which kept me looking healthy and thin. I burned off the carbohydrates with every hard backhand, and I looked good.

The tennis may have given me a National Junior Championship, but it covered up many sins. My junior year of college at Geneva should have been the first warning. I didn't play tennis and couldn't cover up my calories. The free tours of various chocolate factories and the free chocolate at the end of the line that might feed the beast for a week should have been another warning. The thirty extra pounds that I had to work off my senior year was certainly a warning to anyone not addicted to sugar and chocolate. The cravings I experienced were even worse.

Throughout my life, I took antibiotics for every sickness. I trusted doctors to fix whatever was wrong with me. I took whatever antibiotics they prescribed me, and they stopped the symptoms—but never the cause. With each illness, my recovery time grew longer. My immune system weakened with each year. No one in mainstream America knew to ask if diet could affect my health. None of the doctors ever asked me, "What do you put in your mouth?"

Later in life I got married and had two children, my addiction to sugar still thriving. The emotional aspects of a sugar addiction affected my family and me the same way alcoholism affects the families of the alcoholic. Over the years, I experienced depression, anger (some of it directed at my kids), and physical symptoms, all the while not knowing what was causing them.

TIME FOR A CHANGE

Everything finally made sense in 1973 when I attended a health lecture at the Price-Pottenger Nutrition Foundation in San Diego. The lecture explained in detail how sugar upsets the body's chemistry and suppresses the immune system. This lecture changed my life and my health. It also gave me the idea to expand my research into the relationship between minerals in the body and homeostasis, the results of which will be discussed in later chapters.

It was then that I cut sugar out of my diet. Of course, I am admitting to an addiction, so it wasn't a straight line. My progress backslid on more than one occasion and I found myself slipping up more than I would have liked to. I experienced headaches and other withdrawal symptoms. I had to start over after every sugary treat. But as soon as I got on track with my sugar-free lifestyle, I began to see results in as little as a week.

I had received enough information on psychology and analysis over the years to know that if I didn't change my habits, there was a good chance I would pass them on to my children. I knew my kids could grow up to repeat the same cycle of bad diet and bad health that I had lived with up until that point. I dreaded putting my kids on Ritalin or any other drug because of my bad diet.

I began by looking up relevant health and nutrition research. After conducting my own research and continuing to study the information already out there, I earned a PhD in nutrition. I wanted to be able to explain to my kids why sugar really can eventually kill you.

I think I threw myself into my research as a neat way to substitute a more positive addiction, so I could make my dry spells last longer. It was not the yoga (standing on my head to release the phlegm from my chest) that made me feel better. The times when I wasn't eating sugar were the times I felt my best. Somewhere along the way, a majority of my cravings went away, though I keep Altoids around for the ones that do remain. Today, I use them very infrequently.

Just a Sweet Tooth or a Sugar Addiction?

Cooookies! Scarf! Mash! Most of us have grown up hearing these sounds associated with a lovable blue Muppet on Sesame Street, Cookie Monster. Personally, I've waited many years for the Children's Television Workshop to invite me on the show to gently teach Cookie Monster some better nutritional advice, like replacing those cardboard cookies with carrots and eating slowly. So far, I haven't been invited. Oh well, I can dream.

Cookie Monster is a comedic example of sugar as an addictive substance. I had come to believe that Sesame Street would never let Cookie Monster become healthy because the comedic value of a bad example was too great. Imagine my surprise to find that Sesame Street changed the Cookster's tune, just in time for the 2005 season. He now eats cookies in moderation and even advises eating carrots.

What is a Sugar Addiction?

The idea that sugar is an addictive substance is something ordinary people have long assumed to be true, though mainstream science is only beginning to validate those assumptions.

Addiction often includes three steps. First, a person will increase his or her intake of the substance. Next, he or she will experience withdrawal symptoms when access to the substance is cut off. Then, the addict will face an urge to relapse back into using the substance.

Another aspect to the addiction problem is cravings. That intense need for sugar, drugs, or alcohol comes from the body sending out mixed signals, because it may be low in either blood sugar or serotonin. (Serotonin will be explained in the next section.) It could be adrenal fatigue or exhaustion. Sleep deprivation and insomnia also play a role.

The typical response is for the body to send out a "feed me sugar" signal, leading to a desire for sugary snacks, more carbohydrates, or even coffee. The root cause for a sugar craving is the sugar that was eaten in the first place, which unbalanced the body chemistry. I typically tell people to go on Food Plan II or Food Plan III, depending on the severity of the cravings. (See page 111 for Food Plans.)

What Happens in the Body
When We Consume Too Much Sugar?

Addictions pretty much work the same way no matter what the substance is. For example, drugs, alcohol, and sugar all create dependencies in the brain for the substance because without them, the levels of serotonin in the brain drop. Serotonin is a workhorse neurotransmitter and a part of the nervous system that sends nerve impulses to places throughout the body. Addictive substances typically raise serotonin levels for a short period of time, usually resulting in a good, positive feeling. Afterwards the serotonin levels drop—sometimes to levels lower than they were prior to taking the substance—leaving users feeling like they've crashed. Lack of serotonin can also make people feel depressed or blue.

What happens next is the brain senses the drop of serotonin and sends out a "feed me" signal to the body's nervous system that it wants more of whatever made the levels rise in the first place (the addictive substance). Addicts then take in more of the substance, even though with each usage they damage the body's endocrine system, which includes hormones and neurotransmitters. Hormones affect the way the body's organs and tissues function. They are transported to the organs and tissues through bodily fluids, and when people abuse substances, it slows down some of the hormones and speeds up others. The body becomes confused. It eventually gets to the point where it takes more drugs, alcohol, or sugar for an addict to self-medicate the way back to feeling good again.

Dopamine, another neurotransmitter, plays a role in sugar addiction as well. Although you might have had a filling dinner, you may still want a piece of chocolate cake. You don't need this piece of cake to satisfy your hunger, but you want to eat it anyway. The dopamine reward system (which is centered in the brain) gets excited. When a person thinks about that chocolate cake and doesn't eat it, the reward system kicks in and the person becomes depressed or down in the dumps. If the person eats the cake, he or she won't become depressed. The desire to eat the cake overrides the fact that you are not hungry, leading you to consume tasty foods even when you're full. Thanks to dopamine, we do not always have the ability to say no to these tasty foods.

Eating sugar may feel good and people can develop mental processes designed to get more of it until they learn to live without it. Once a behavior becomes set, it often takes therapy and support to help break the cycle until some time passes and the body doesn't need the substance so much.

Statistics and Studies on Sugar Addiction

Scientists began thinking of sugar as an addictive substance in the 1980s. They always felt that people normally have sugar in their bodies, so how could we be addicted to it? All the carbohydrates we eat are broken down into simple sugars. The protein and fat we consume also partially break down into simple sugar. So, the body always has some sugar in it. For many years, I have felt differently about sugar addiction. There was no doubt in my mind that I had seen people who were addicted to sugar. Some knew that they were and did not want to be. Many asked for help.

Finally, someone funded proper research. At the beginning of the twenty-first century, Dr. Nicole Avena, a researcher at Princeton University, and her associates began studying sugar addiction. One of their studies was performed on rats, who were fed a diet of sugar. When given the choice between sugar and healthy food, the rats pushed the healthy food away because they wanted nothing but sugar. When the rats were given a choice between plain water and sugar water, they chose the sugar water. Taking the sugar water away caused the rats to experience withdrawal symptoms. The researchers found that the rats who went cold turkey experienced shakes and chattering teeth, symptoms common to those experienced by humans crashing from a drug high. When the rats were given the choice between regular and sugar water again, they continued to pull the lever that fed them sugar.

Another study was done at the University of Bordeaux in France, where Magalie Lenoir and her associates compared the relative response of saccharin (a sugar substitute) and cocaine. The reason they picked a sugar substitute over sugar was because they did not want the calories in sugar to be part of the equation. A rat might have chosen sugar to fill its stomach rather than for sugar's sweetness. The rats were given the option to choose between intravenous cocaine and water sweetened with saccharin. The large majority of the rats (94 percent) preferred the saccharin. Even in cases when the rat was addicted to cocaine first and then given the choice between cocaine and saccharin, it chose saccharin. The researchers concluded that the sweetness of sugar (and its substitutes) can surpass cocaine rewards, even in addicts.

Essentially, the studies indicate that sweetness may have been the original addiction, since drugs and alcohol use the same neurons that are related to food consumption. Originally, getting a good feeling from a food was thought to have motivated the cavemen to get more food necessary for survival. Naturally, sweet foods like whole fruit can spike a hunter-gatherer's calorie intake so that he wouldn't die between animals killed. However, we now live in a world where food is plentiful—well beyond the tolerances created by that original diet.

As you can see, sugar is not a simple addiction. It is readily accepted in our food supply and in our life, and the temptation is there on a continual basis. It is quite possible this is why this addiction is so hard to break.

Sugar addiction is also evident in the official sugar consumption data from the U.S. Government. The government first started recording sugar consumption in 1966. That year, the average person consumed 116 pounds of sugar. The highest recorded consumption was in 1999 at 151 pounds per person.

It has since dropped to around 142 pounds per person per year, which equals about 24 teaspoons or $1/2$ cup of sugar per day.[1] However, this slight drop doesn't even begin to reverse the many years of dramatic increases.

How to Tell if You Have a Sugar Addiction

Now, let's talk about you. Do you have an addiction to sugar? Perhaps you do and you simply haven't realized it yet. Consider what you eat on a daily basis. How much of what you consume contains sugar or sweeteners? How long can you go without the major sources of sugar in your diet?

Think about it. Do you drink one, two, three, or four sodas per day? With what sweeteners do you cut your morning coffee? Do you use sugar? Honey? What about the morning doughnut that goes with the coffee? After each meal do you need to have something sweet? Are most of your snacks sugar-laden?

If you consume sugar every day from one or more of these sources there is a good chance that you may have a sugar addiction problem. If that is the case, remember—you are not alone.

Cooookie! Cooookie! It may be fun and cute for a blue puppet to crave sweets like that, but it's terrible when anyone else does it.

SUGAR BY ANY OTHER NAME IS JUST AS TROUBLESOME

Before I go into detail about my research and the results it yielded, I think it is important to provide a basic definition of exactly what sugar is. Sugar is a food carbohydrate that is interpreted by the human taste buds as sweet. Refer to the following list to see the different types of sugar discussed throughout the book.

Sugar in its Many Forms

- Agave syrup or nectar
- Barley malt
- Beet sugar
- Brown sugar
- Cane sugar
- Cane syrup
- Confections sugar
- Crystalline fructose
- Date sugar
- Evaporated sugarcane
- Fructose
- Fruit juice concentrate
- Galactose
- Glucose
- Granulated sugar
- High fructose corn syrup
- Honey
- Invert sugar
- Lactose
- Liquid cane sugar or syrup
- Maltose
- Maple syrup
- Molasses
- Powdered sugar
- Raw sugar
- Rice syrup
- Sugarcane syrup
- Table sugar
- Turbinado sugar
- Unrefined sugar
- White sugar

My research led me to discover that sugar is one of the many stressors that throws the human body chemistry out of the balance we call homeostasis, a word you will hear more about as you read this book.

As mentioned, Americans consume sugar and other similar sweeteners at an average of 48 teaspoons per person per day. The next useful thing to know is how low the body's threshold for added sugar really is. For most healthy people, it is about 2 teaspoons of added sugar at one time, two or three times a day. Is it any wonder that commonly quoted statistics about overweight people and obesity say scary things like 62 percent of adults are overweight (and that half of those people are obese)?

During my research process, I began conducting private consultations. Nearly every blood test that I took of a sick person showed various mineral imbalances within the body. The patients' histories usually revealed an extremely high correlation between diet, psychological situation, exercise, and spiritual life as well.

CONCLUSION

Everybody who hasn't sold out to Big Sugar has some understanding that less sugar is good and almost none is better. It is difficult to eliminate sugar from your diet, since it is in many recipes and is used as a cheap filler in many processed foods. For this reason, I have developed three food plans to help get sugar intake down to a reasonable and healthy amount. There are also recipes to help you along your way to a sugarless diet. You can find these plans and recipes later in this book, in Chapter 7 (page 107).

I have learned to put up with the small amount of high fructose corn syrup in ketchup. But I can't remember the last time I had a hot fudge sundae or an Oreo cookie. Overcoming my addiction is an ongoing process I take one day at a time, all the while enjoying the differences between being sick all the time, not wanting to look in the mirror, and being angry or depressed to being sick infrequently, not minding what I see in the mirror, and waking up and going to bed happy.

Eliminating sugar from my diet has changed me for the better. The proof is in the pudding of my life. I'm a woman in my 70s and I still do the things I like to do. I am a grandmother to my two energetic grandchildren, and I also play tennis, go hiking, lecture, and travel to developing countries.

I can't claim to be the first person to speak out against sugar, because I couldn't have learned what my problem was without finding the books and journal articles written by the giants upon whose shoulders I stand. I do, however, pride myself in knowing that I was in the game early on, before doctors started to join the bandwagon.

I wrote this book to balance my new research and information with the data that is tried and true. My opinion over the years has been unwavering, but research has led to new developments and information to back up my point.

Health or sickness—you choose.

By the way, I noticed a "hot buy" in a flyer from my local drug-store—5 pounds of C&H granulated sugar for $1.99. That's about forty cents a pound. That may be the cheapest food you can buy. The sugar industry has great lobbyists, so of course, the government sub-sidizes sugar. Nonsense. However, I must admit that if it were 1970, I would have run to the store to buy 10 pounds, but since I know now what sugar does to my body, forget it.

2

---

140 Reasons Why Sugar is Ruining Your Health

For about twenty years I have been collecting "Reasons Why Sugar Is Ruining Your Health."

I have found them in everything from the Harvard medical publication *HEALTHbeat* to just perusing the web. They are difficult to find and many times more difficult to read because of medical jargon. I feel that the long-term use of added sugar can be a problem for many people and can cause many diseases.

Join me twenty years from now and I will probably have many more reasons.

1. Sugar can suppress the immune system.

2. Sugar upsets the mineral relationships in the body.

3. Sugar can cause juvenile delinquency in children.

4. Sugar eaten during pregnancy and lactation can influence muscle force production in offspring, which can affect an individual's ability to exercise.

5. Sugar in soda, when consumed by children, results in the children drinking less milk.

6. Sugar can elevate glucose and insulin responses and return them to fasting levels slower in oral contraceptive users.

7. Sugar can increase reactive oxygen species (ROS), which damage cells and tissues.

8. Sugar can cause hyperactivity, anxiety, inability to concentrate, and crankiness in children.

9. Sugar can produce a significant rise in triglycerides.

10. Sugar reduces the body's ability to defend against bacterial infection.

11. Sugar causes a decline in tissue elasticity and function—the more sugar you eat, the more elasticity and function you lose.

12. Sugar reduces high-density lipoproteins (HDL).

13. Sugar can lead to chromium deficiency.

14. Sugar can lead to ovarian cancer.

15. Sugar can increase fasting levels of glucose.

16. Sugar causes copper deficiency.

17. Sugar interferes with the body's absorption of calcium and magnesium.

18. Sugar may make eyes more vulnerable to age-related macular degeneration.

19. Sugar raises the level of neurotransmitters: dopamine, serotonin, and norepinephrine.

20. Sugar can cause hypoglycemia.

21. Sugar can lead to an acidic digestive tract.

22. Sugar can cause a rapid rise of adrenaline levels in children.

23. Sugar is frequently malabsorbed in patients with functional bowel disease.

24. Sugar can cause premature aging.

25. Sugar can lead to alcoholism.

26. Sugar can cause tooth decay.

27. Sugar can lead to obesity.

28. Sugar increases the risk of Crohn's disease and ulcerative colitis.

29. Sugar can cause gastric or duodenal ulcers.

30. Sugar can cause arthritis.

31. Sugar can cause learning disorders in school children.

32. Sugar assists the uncontrolled growth of Candida Albicans (yeast infections).

33. Sugar can cause gallstones.

34. Sugar can cause heart disease.

35. Sugar can cause appendicitis.

36. Sugar can cause hemorrhoids.

37. Sugar can cause varicose veins.

38. Sugar can lead to periodontal disease.

39. Sugar can contribute to osteoporosis.

40. Sugar contributes to saliva acidity.

41. Sugar can cause a decrease in insulin sensitivity.

42. Sugar can lower the amount of Vitamin E in the blood.

43. Sugar can decrease the amount of growth hormones in the body.

44. Sugar can increase cholesterol.

45. Sugar increases advanced glycation end products (AGEs), which form when sugar binds non-enzymatically to protein.

46. Sugar can interfere with the absorption of protein.

47. Sugar causes food allergies.

48. Sugar can contribute to diabetes.

49. Sugar can cause toxemia during pregnancy.

50. Sugar can lead to eczema in children.

51. Sugar can cause cardiovascular disease.

52. Sugar can impair the structure of DNA.

53. Sugar can change the structure of protein.

54. Sugar can make the skin wrinkle by changing the structure of collagen.

55. Sugar can cause cataracts.

56. Sugar can cause emphysema.

57. Sugar can cause atherosclerosis.

58. Sugar can promote an elevation of low-density lipoproteins (LDL).

59. Sugar can impair the physiological homeostasis of many systems in the body.

60. Sugar lowers enzymes' ability to function.

61. Sugar intake is associated with the development of Parkinson's disease.

62. Sugar can increase the size of the liver by making the liver cells divide.

63. Sugar can increase the amount of liver fat.

64. Sugar can increase kidney size and produce pathological changes in the kidney.

65. Sugar can damage the pancreas.

66. Sugar can increase the body's fluid retention.

67. Sugar is the number one enemy of the bowel movement.

68. Sugar can cause myopia (nearsightedness).

69. Sugar can compromise the lining of the capillaries.

70. Sugar can make tendons more brittle.

71. Sugar can cause headaches, including migraines.

72. Sugar plays a role in pancreatic cancer in women.

73. Sugar can adversely affect children's grades in school.

74. Sugar can cause depression.

75. Sugar increases the risk of gastric cancer.

76. Sugar can cause dyspepsia (indigestion).

77. Sugar can increase the risk of developing gout.

78. Sugar can increase the levels of glucose in the blood much higher than complex carbohydrates in a glucose tolerance test can.

79. Sugar reduces learning capacity.

80. Sugar can cause two blood proteins—albumin and lipoproteins—to function less effectively, which may reduce the body's ability to handle fat and cholesterol.

81. Sugar can contribute to Alzheimer's disease.

82. Sugar can cause platelet adhesiveness, which causes blood clots.

83. Sugar can cause hormonal imbalance—some hormones become underactive and others become overactive.

84. Sugar can lead to the formation of kidney stones.

85. Sugar can cause free radicals and oxidative stress.

86. Sugar can lead to biliary tract cancer.

87. Sugar increases the risk of pregnant adolescents delivering a small-for-gestational-age (SGA) infant.

88. Sugar can lead to a substantial decrease in the length of pregnancy among adolescents.

89. Sugar slows food's travel time through the gastrointestinal tract.

90. Sugar increases the concentration of bile acids in stool and bacterial enzymes in the colon, which can modify bile to produce cancer-causing compounds and colon cancer.

91. Sugar increases estradiol (the most potent form of naturally occurring estrogen) in men.

92. Sugar combines with and destroys phosphatase, an enzyme, which makes digestion more difficult.

93. Sugar can be a risk factor for gallbladder cancer.

94. Sugar is an addictive substance.

95. Sugar can be intoxicating, similar to alcohol.

96. Sugar can aggravate premenstrual syndrome (PMS).

97. Sugar can decrease emotional stability.

98. Sugar promotes excessive food intake in obese people.

99. Sugar can worsen the symptoms of children with attention deficit disorder (ADD).

100. Sugar can slow the ability of the adrenal glands to function.

101. Sugar can cut off oxygen to the brain when given to people intravenously.

102. Sugar is a risk factor for lung cancer.

103. Sugar increases the risk of polio.

104. Sugar can cause epileptic seizures.

105. Sugar can increase systolic blood pressure (pressure when heart is contracting).

106. Sugar can induce cell death.

107. Sugar can increase the amount of food that you eat.

108. Sugar can cause antisocial behavior in juvenile delinquents.

109. Sugar can lead to prostate cancer.

110. Sugar dehydrates newborns.

111. Sugar can cause women to give birth to babies with low birth weight.

112. Sugar is associated with a worse outcome of schizophrenia.

113. Sugar can raise homocysteine levels in the bloodstream.

114. Sugar increases the risk of breast cancer.

115. Sugar is a risk factor in small intestine cancer.

116. Sugar can cause laryngeal cancer.

117. Sugar induces salt and water retention.

118. Sugar can contribute to mild memory loss.

119. Sugar water, when given to children shortly after birth, results in those children preferring sugar water to regular water throughout childhood.

120. Sugar causes constipation.

121. Sugar can cause brain decay in pre-diabetic and diabetic women.

122. Sugar can increase the risk of stomach cancer.

123. Sugar can cause metabolic syndrome.

124. Sugar increases neural tube defects in embryos when it is consumed by pregnant women.

125. Sugar can cause asthma.

126. Sugar increases the chances of getting irritable bowel syndrome.

127. Sugar can affect central reward systems.

128. Sugar can cause cancer of the rectum.

129. Sugar can cause endometrial cancer.

130. Sugar can cause renal (kidney) cell cancer.

131. Sugar can cause liver tumors.

132. Sugar can increase inflammatory markers in the bloodstreams of overweight people.

133. Sugar plays a role in the cause and the continuation of acne.

134. Sugar can ruin the sex life of both men and women by turning off the gene that controls the sex hormones.

135. Sugar can cause fatigue, moodiness, nervousness, and depression.

136. Sugar can make many essential nutrients less available to cells.

137. Sugar can increase uric acid in blood.

138. Sugar can lead to higher C-peptide concentrations.

139. Sugar causes inflammation.

140. Sugar can cause diverticulitis, a small bulging sac pushing outward from the colon wall that is inflammed.*

For each reason's citation, see Notes on page 151.

Now that you're aware of what sugar is doing to your body, it's time to explore in further detail how and why it is slowly killing you.

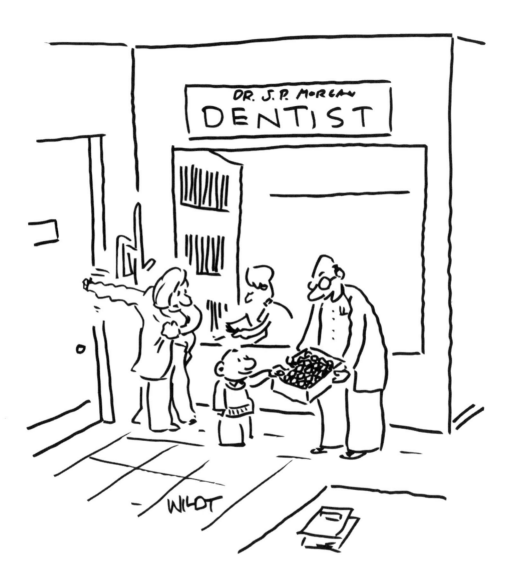

"Another cavity-free visit for Timmy.
Have a candy...take the whole box!"

3

Homeostasis: The Balance in the Body

The reason I am writing about homeostasis in *Suicide by Sugar* is because homeostasis relates to sugar in a big way. This will become self-evident as the story on homeostasis unfolds.

Walter B. Cannon, PhD, MD (1871–1945), a Harvard professor, coined the word "homeostasis" in his brilliant 1932 book, *The Wisdom of the Body*. Cannon graduated from Harvard cum laude, and was head of the physiology department there for many years. Also, Cannon was the first to understand that carbohydrates go through the digestive tract the fastest, that protein is next, and that fat takes the longest time to get through. For his understanding of the body and where disease comes from, he is my unsung hero. (To find out where you can get Cannon's book, see Recommended Reading, page 149.)

On a side note, this brilliant man also discovered the "fight or flight" response.

BALANCE DOES NOT MEAN A CANDY BAR IN EACH HAND

For people, homeostasis commonly refers to the internal balance of the body's electro-magnetic and chemical systems. This balance permits and encourages proper performance of the internal functions necessary for growth, healing, and life itself. Our bodies heal when we are in homeostasis.

The difference between a sick person and a healthy person is the person's ability to gain and maintain homeostasis. Sick people have a difficult time doing this. When our bodies cannot maintain homeostasis over a period of time, we get sick. Each person is different, so

21

the number of sicknesses a person will get, how long the illnesses will last, and how severe the illnesses are will vary on an individual basis. Some of the items that determine this are your genetic blueprint, how much sugar and other abusive foods you eat, what role distress has played in your life, your exposure to chemicals, and other factors. There are many things that upset body chemistry and throw us out of homeostasis on a daily basis, sugar being one of the main ones. This assertion applies to both degenerative diseases and infectious diseases.

SUGAR CAN THROW OFF HOMEOSTASIS

There are many systems within the human body that help regulate homeostasis. The endocrine system, which releases hormones into the bloodstream, is the primary regulator. The main endocrine glands are the pancreas, adrenal glands, male and female glands, hypothalamus, pituitary glands, and thyroid glands. Each one of these glands secretes hormones into the bloodstream to help regulate homeostasis.

When sugar is ingested, the first gland to feel its impact is the pancreas. After sugar injestion the blood sugar rises, and the pancreas secretes insulin. The main reason the insulin is secreted is to bring the blood sugar level down, back to homeostasis. When we eat more sugar than our pancreas can handle, the pancreas becomes exhausted and can, in turn, secrete too much insulin or not enough insulin. If the pancreas secretes too much insulin, the blood is not able to get enough sugar. This can lead to hypoglycemia (low blood sugar). Consequently, if the pancreas doesn't secrete enough insulin, our blood will absorb too much sugar, which can lead to hyperglycemia (high blood sugar) or diabetes.

All the glands work together. When the pancreas is struggling, some of the glands come to its aid, and they start secreting too much or too little of their hormones into the bloodstream in an attempt to regain and maintain homeostasis. This can throw the whole endocrine system into disarray, causing some of the glands to become depleted. This is the reason that so many of us have hypoglycemia, diabetes, thyroid problems, and adrenal exhaustion. It's also the reason women have menopausal problems. Yes, excess sugar can do all of that.

Minerals:
Yes, They Are Important

No mineral is an island. Minerals can only function in relation to each other. (See Figure 3.1 on page 24). If one mineral drops in the bloodstream, the other minerals will not function as well. When we consume too much sugar, our bodies are forced to readjust their composition to make up for the excess amounts of glucose and fructose. In order to do this, minerals are pulled from the bloodstream. The minerals that are left do not function as well as they should in the absence of the ones that were pulled. Needless to say, in this type of situation, the body's chemistry has been thrown off.

Minerals are needed by many of the body's systems. The endocrine system, immune system, and digestive system all need minerals to function properly. Enzymes, which help us digest food, need particular minerals to work optimally. When there are not enough functioning minerals in the bloodstream, the immune system's phagocytes become depleted. Any substance in the body that can't be used is automatically treated as a toxin. This includes unused minerals.[1,2] Toxic calcium, for instance, can cause tooth plaque, kidney stones, arthritis, cataracts, bone spurs, hardening of the arteries, and many other maladies.

Calcium and phosphorus give our bodies structure through the formation of bones and teeth. Other minerals initiate a reaction in enzyme systems, our cells, and our body fluids. This helps our bodies grow, maintain, and regulate themselves. It also provides us with energy. A slight change from the normal mineral composition in the cells can have extreme effects on the body, even if the actual mineral makeup of the body as a whole has not changed all that drastically.[3]

One such effect the body can suffer is that enzymes within the body won't function as well as they should. Earlier, you learned that enzymes need minerals to function optimally. Enzymes are proteins created by the body that speed up body processes. For example, enzymes play a very important role in the digestive process. Digestive enzymes break food into its simplest components: carbohydrates into simple sugars, fat into fatty acids, and proteins into amino acids. When the enzymes cannot function well due to a deficiency in minerals, not all of the food is properly digested. Undigested protein, for example, can get into the bloodstream in the form of polypeptides, which are very small protein molecules that contain amino acids.[4,5]

In his book *Brain Allergies,* Dr. William Philpott writes, "One of the most important systemic functions of the pancreas is to supply proteolytic enzymes, which act as regulatory mechanisms over inflammatory reactions in the body."[6] Proteolytic enzymes are from the pancreas and aid in the digestion of proteins into amino acids. The improper digestion of proteins can be caused by insufficient pancreatic proteolytic enzymes. As a result, unusable protein molecules are absorbed into the blood, reaching body tissues in their partially digested forms. This is called the leaky gut syndrome, or gut permeability. Since they are only partially digested, the body treats them as invaders, which can cause toxicity and inflammation in different organs or tissues within the body.

MINERAL WHEEL

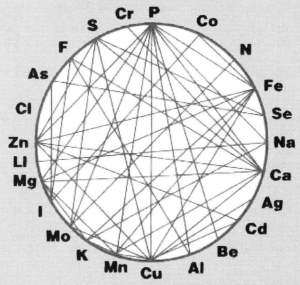

Minerals work only in relation to each other.

FIGURE 3.1   THE MINERAL WHEEL.

The partially-digested protein and other undigested foods are usually in particles too large to be used by the cells. Thus, they may get into the bloodstream and cause a food allergy, which would eventually cause havoc in the bloodstream.[7] When I say food allergy, I do mean the classic symptoms of an allergy—runny eyes, sinusitis, sneezing, and a scratchy throat.[8,9] Alternately, these particles can go to the joints, tissues, or bones and cause arthritis.[10,11] They can also go to the body's nervous system and cause multiple sclerosis (MS), a disease varying in severity.[12] Some MS sufferers experience mild symptoms, such as numbness in the limbs, while others may experience more severe ailments, such as paralysis or blindness.

Medical research also shows that this foreign matter can go into the skin and cause hives, eczema, and psoriasis (a skin condition consisting of gray or silvery flaky patches on the skin, which is red and inflamed).[13,14,15] Ulcerative colitis (a disease involving inflammation of the inner lining of the colon and rectum) and Crohn's disease (a disease involving inflammation anywhere in the digestive tract from the mouth to the rectum) can also be caused by partially digested protein.[16] Essentially, this unusable protein can go anywhere in the blood and cause problems.

Unfortunately, it isn't just the partially digested food particles that can get into the bloodstream. Sometimes the enzymes that do not work properly slip into the bloodstream as well, causing the cells to become toxic.[17] Neither partially digested food nor digestive enzymes belong in the bloodstream. They only belong in the digestive tract. When this happens, our immune system looks at the undigested or partially digested food and enzymes as foreign invaders and comes to the defense.[18,19] Remember, this partially digested and undigested food is present in the body as a result of consuming too much sugar.

To fight back, the body's white blood cells (the primary element of the immune system) need a regular supply of properly digested protein. The strain on the body's enzymes caused by excess sugar (among other factors) results in a less functional immune system that is less able to defend against the diseases floating around the environment. There is a complex interplay between what we eat, the stress in our life, environmental factors, and our own genetic blueprint. Each one of these criteria help determine our body's ability to regain and maintain homeostasis.

Sugar suppresses the immune system. It depletes levels of phagocytes (the white blood cells that are needed for strong immune function and that eat up harmful bacteria) and this reduces the body's ability to fight infection and disease.

The makeup of our blood needs to stay balanced in order for us to remain in homoeostasis. For this to happen, the elements in our blood are constantly readjusting themselves within a very narrow range. One of the elements in our blood that does just this is glucose. Thus, consuming too much sugar is one of the main ways people can upset their body chemistry, throwing it out of homeostasis.

Sugar is an acid-forming food. Therefore, our bodies can become acidic when we eat sugar. But, our bodies do not like this acidic state, so they pull minerals (like calcium, magnesium, and phosphorus) from the bloodstream, trying to become alkaline again; trying to regain and maintain homeostasis.

Doctors and clinicians don't usually test the total blood chemistry of a person before and after he or she eats sugar. If they did, they would find that minerals can increase, decrease, and generally change their working relationship with each other. According to my own research, I have found that this can happen when a person consumes as little as two teaspoons of sugar at one time.

SUGAR'S UNBALANCING ACT

I have focused most of this chapter on sugar, but there are other lifestyle factors that can knock our bodies out of homeostasis. One of these is our emotional state. Therefore, feeling sad, angry, or anxious can affect our balanced body chemistry and ultimately have the same effect that consuming sugar would have.[20,21]

However, the main culprit here is sugar, simply because we consume way too much of it for our bodies to handle. We evolved from early man, whose diet was raw and cooked meat, fat, scavenged foods and vegetables, seeds, and clean water. Our bodies have not evolved beyond being able to eat this low-sugar Neolithic diet, as indicated by my research. Two teaspoons of sugar (in any of its forms) at one time seems to be the limit of what most healthy people can handle. As for sick people, I don't think their bodies can handle any sugar.

When we eat sugar, our bodies can only respond in one way. They must adjust and try to rebalance themselves after each sugary insult. This balancing act pulls minerals from the body where they are needed and messes up body chemistry, eventually making us sick. Considering the amount of sugar we eat, our bodies do not have the digestive mechanisms to handle the glut of sugar that we consume on a daily basis.

We create our own illnesses with every sugary treat we consume and every angry thought we experience. Most people don't know what they're doing to their bodies, because homeostasis is hard to test for. For you, this will change. You have more information now, and there is also a kit designed to test for homeostasis, the acid alkaline balance, and excess calcium in the urine (see page 182 for more on this kit). Keep your body in homeostasis and it will heal and stay healthy.

CONCLUSION

As you can see, the body is like an orchestra. All the parts have to play in harmony in an orchestra, just as all the parts in a body must play in harmony for the body to function optimally. As there is an orchestra leader, you are the leader of your body. You decide what you eat, think, say, feel, and do—and all of these actions can affect your body chemistry. In an orchestra, if one violin is out of tune there are problems. In your body, if one mineral is out of balance it affects the whole body. So, you can direct your body in harmony or in discourse, just like an orchestra leader can do. I highly suggest you keep harmony with your body by making the right choices.

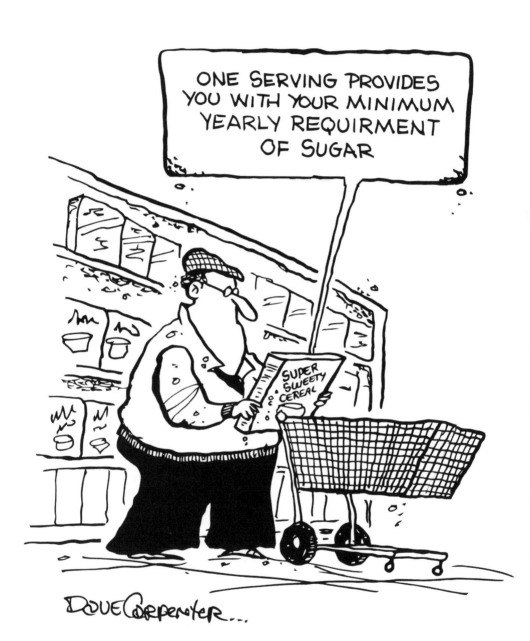

4

What Sugar Can Do to Your Blood Glucose Is No Sweet Matter

T his chapter will tell you about what happens to your blood glucose (sugar) when you eat carbohydrates, with an emphasis on sugar. I hope you will read this chapter closely as there is information in here that is usually not mentioned when a person is reading about blood glucose.

First you will learn about the glycemic index (GI) and the glycemic load (GL). Then you will find out that when choosing which carbohydrates to eat, you should base your decision on much more than just the GI and GL. I believe these measurements have been misused, and I hope you will get a better picture of how to choose healthy carbohydrates other than using the GI and GL.

The last part of the chapter concerns the oral glucose tolerance test (OGTT). I hope to show you there are alternatives to this invasive test that can give similar results.

GLYCEMIC INDEX AND GLYCEMIC LOAD

When considering blood glucose levels, determining how high a person's blood glucose goes when he or she eats a carbohydrate is only one of the two factors that must be taken into consideration. The other is the amount, or quantity, of the carbohydrate that is being consumed. This is why scientists came up with glycemic index and glycemic load.

Glycemic Index

The GI is a numerical system of measuring how quickly a food triggers a rise in blood glucose. GI ranks foods according to their effect on blood glucose levels. This index is usually based on an amount of food that contains 50 grams of carbohydrates, and is given a number. The higher the number, the quicker the glucose response will be. Foods with a low GI break down slowly, so the glucose in the food is released gradually. This will cause a small rise in blood glucose. High GI foods break down quicker, so the glucose is released in a surge, which can trigger a dramatic spike in blood sugar.

GI is calculated by feeding specific foods to people and tracking the body's response. As mentioned, GI is based on 50 grams of carbohydrates. It's important to understand that in order to get 50 grams of carbohydrates, larger quantities of a food must be consumed. Foods that are low in carbohydrates will need to be consumed in greater quantities to get the 50 grams needed to test for GI.

To calculate GI, an amount of food containing 50 grams of carbohydrates is fed to eight to ten people. Over the next two hours, the blood glucose levels of the test subjects are checked every fifteen to thirty minutes. This entire process is repeated two or three times. The blood sugar level values of the test subjects are averaged and compared to a standard food, usually pure glucose (which has an arbitrary GI of 100).

Some foods are not tested for GI because you would have to eat too much of them in order to get the 50 grams of carbohydrates needed. These foods, when eaten alone, may not cause a significant rise in blood glucose, but this doesn't mean they're healthy. They may contain large amounts of fat or calories, neither of which is good for you.

Eating larger quantities of a food won't cause its GI to go up, because the GI indicates the food's ranking compared to other foods with the same amount of carbohydrates. The GI measures how quickly the carbohydrate triggers a rise in blood glucose. It does not measure how high the blood glucose actually goes. For example, if a food has a GI of 25, no matter how much of that food you eat, its GI will still be 25. All this means is that regardless of the quantity you eat the food in, the rate at which it triggers a rise in blood glucose remains the same. Of course, the more of the food you eat, the higher the resulting blood glucose will be—but the rate at which the blood glucose increases will remain the same. When it comes to serving size, that's where GL comes into play.

Glycemic Load

The GL is a method of assessing the impact of carbohydrate consumption. It takes GI into account, but provides a fuller picture than the GI does alone. The GL is more valuable—it gives a number based on the amount of carbohydrates in a serving, rather than the amount of food it takes to get 50 grams of carbohydrates. This is good because many times, a person doesn't eat 50 grams of carbohydrates at once. It would be difficult to eat 50 grams of carbohydrates from watermelon or carrots, although both have a high GI.

GL is calculated by multiplying a food's GI by the amount of carbohydrates (in grams) in the serving. This number is then divided by 100 to get the GL. For example, a slice of watermelon with a GI of 72 and a carbohydrate content of 5 grams would have a GL of 3.6 (GI [72] x carbohydrate content [5] = 360 ÷ 100 = 3.6). A GL of 3.6 is very low.

The usefulness of GL is based on the idea that consuming a high GI food in small quantities (resulting in fewer grams of carbohydrates) would have the same effect on blood sugar as consuming a low GI food in larger quantities. For example, a food with a GI of 100 and a carbohydrate content of 10 grams has a GL of 10 (GI [100] x carbohydrate content [10] = 1,000 ÷ 100 = 10). A food with a GI of 10 and 100 grams of carbohydrates also has a GL of 10 (GI [10] x carbohydrate content [100] = 1,000 ÷ 100 = 10).

Example of GI and GL in Carrots

A good reason to consider the GL of a food is the example of carrots. Carrots have a high GI based on the 50 grams of carbohydrates needed to test for GI. However, there are only three or four grams of carbohydrates in an individual carrot. To get the 50 grams needed to yield the high GI, you would need to eat nearly 3 cups of carrots (or nearly 15 whole carrots). The average person does not eat this many carrots in one sitting, so the amount of carbohydrates in the carrots actually eaten would be low. By considering both GI and serving size, GL gives a more realistic depiction of how the food you eat will affect your blood glucose levels.

What to Consider When Choosing a Carbohydrate to Eat

While GI and GL are both useful tools for determining how a food will affect your blood sugar, they both fail to take into account many items that are important when you eat a food. It is necessary to know both GI and GL to understand a food's effect on blood sugar, but even then there are flaws in the bigger picture. When choosing a food, it is far more important to think of the following items than to think of the GI and GL. Neither GI nor GL take into account the following:

- Nutrient value, such as the vitamins and minerals contained in specific foods.

- How the food affects the immune system, the endocrine system, the digestive system, the liver, and the minerals.

- The fact that most sugars, fruits, and vegetables are made up of glucose and fructose. The fructose in a product does not raise blood glucose, but the glucose does. For example, table sugar, maple sugar, honey, and fruits and vegetables have about 50 percent glucose and 50 percent fructose. Products made from corn can be modified as to how much glucose and fructose they contain (the number is usually 55 percent glucose and 45 percent fructose, but the amount of fructose can go higher). Since fructose doesn't raise blood glucose, foods containing fructose may have low GIs and GLs—but they are not necessarily healthy.

- The fact that when a high GI food is eaten with fat or protein, the blood glucose level stays in a normal range. For example, when a potato is eaten with butter or sour cream and some protein (like meat, fish, or soy), the blood glucose becomes normally elevated. The fat and protein stabilize the starch in the potato, because fat and protein travel slower through the body. We established earlier that carbohydrates go through the system fastest, then protein, then fat.

- The total amount of sugar in a product. GI and GL only consider the amount of carbohydrates. Total sugar is important, since all forms of sugar can upset the body chemistry, deplete the minerals, and suppress the immune system.

- Whether a food is a whole food or a processed food. The fact is that whole foods normally have higher nutritional values than processed foods. For example, when you need a quick source of energy, choosing the appropriate whole food might provide you a higher level of GI and GL, but it will be without the problems inherent in processed foods.

- Satiety factor. Do you feel full after you eat? Many times a high glycemic food has sugar in it. Sugar is addictive and makes you want more, because you do not feel full after you eat it. A potato with a high GI is filling and makes you feel satisfied. Isn't it better to feel satisfied rather than to want more?

- The calorie count. Many times a food is low in GI and GL but has a high calorie count. Apples have a GI of 38 (as shown in Table 4.2 on page 35), and a medium-size apple, weighing 138 grams, provides a GL of 6. This is a low GL, and most would consider the apple to be a very appropriate snack. But now look at peanuts. A 1-ounce (28 gram) serving of peanuts not only weighs less than the apple, but has a much lower GI (14), and provides an even lower GL (1). Based on GL alone, you would have to believe that a 1-ounce serving of peanuts was a better dietary choice than an apple. But if you take a look at the calories contained in these two foods, you'll see that the apple contains approximately 65 calories, while 1 ounce of peanuts contains about 164 calories.

If this sounds confusing, it certainly is—even for me. Sometimes, a visual aid helps. Table 4.1 and Table 4.2 will give you some more information that I hope will clear a few things up.

Beverage	Portion Size (grams)	Portion Size (fl. oz.)	Calories	GI*	GL†	Carbs (grams)	Sugar (grams)	Sugar (tsps)
TABLE 4.1 NUTRITIONAL VALUES FOR CERTAIN BEVERAGES								
Apple juice, unsweetened	250 g	8 oz.	117	40	12	29 g	28 g	7 tsp.
Coca-Cola	250 g	8 oz.	120	63	16	26 g	26 g	6½ tsp.
Ensure Plus	252 g	8 oz.	350	44	22	50 g	50 g	12½ tsp.
Orange juice	250 g	8 oz.	112	50	13	26 g	26 g	6½ tsp.

*GI values can be classified into three levels—low (ranging from 1 to 55), medium (ranging from 56 to 69), and high (ranging from 70 to 100).

†GL values can be classified into three levels—low (ranging from 1 to 10), medium (ranging from 11 to 19), and high (20 and above).

If you were not confused before, these tables might send you to the next chapter fast. This was difficult information for me to get and to understand. You will see the notes at the end of the book. I had to hop from one to another to get this information.

Here is some important information about Table 4.1 and Table 4.2:

- All values in the tables are approximate.

- The difference between an apple and apple juice. The GI is basically the same for both, but the GL for a whole apple is about half the GL of an 8-ounce serving of apple juice. Basically, what this means is both the apple and the apple juice will elevate blood glucose at the same rate—but the GL of the apple juice shows that the juice is far worse for you than the apple. The sugar content of apple juice is almost double that of an apple. This is similar for grapes and oranges when compared to grape juice and orange juice. So, eat your fruit whole.

	TABLE 4.2 NUTRITIONAL VALUES FOR CERTAIN FOODS							
Food	**Portion Size (grams)**	**Portion Size (fl. oz.)**	**Calories**	**GI***	**GL†**	**Carbs (grams)**	**Sugar (grams)**	**Sugar (tsps)**
Agave Nectar	12 g	2 tsp.	40	27	3	12 g	12 g	3 tsp.
Apple with skin	120 g	1 medium apple	65	38	6	16 g	12 g	3 tsp.
Carrots	72 g	1 large carrot	30	47	3	7 g	3 g	¾ tsp.
Cashew nuts	28 g	1 oz.	160	25	3	13 g	2 g	½ tsp.
Corn kernels	150 g	¾ cup	134	60	20	33 g	4 g	1 tsp.
Grapes	120 g	1 cup	35	42	7	18 g	17 g	4½ tsp.
Ice cream, vanilla	72 g	½ cup	145	62	8	17 g	15 g	3¾ tsp.
M&M's	56 g	2 oz.	295	68	29	43 g	38 g	9½ tsp.
Peanuts	28 g	1 oz.	164	14	1	6 g	4 g	1 tsp.
Pinto beans, boiled	150 g	¾ cup	230	39	1	3 g	0	0
Popcorn	20 g	2 cups	110	89	12	13 g	0	0
Potato, baked, with skin	150 g	1 medium potato	115	85	23	27 g	4 g	1 tsp.
Rice, white, boiled	150 g	1 cup	205	64	23	36 g	0 g	0
Sucrose (table sugar)	10 g	2 tsp.	38	68	7	10 g	8 g	2 tsp.
Sweet potato	150 g	¾ cup	135	48	17	36 g	15 g	3¾ tsp.
Watermelon, sliced	240 g	1 cup	52	72	4	5 g	4 g	1 tsp.

*GI values can be classified into three levels—low (ranging from 1 to 55), medium (ranging from 56 to 69), and high (ranging from 70 to 100).

†GL values can be classified into three levels—low (ranging from 1 to 10), medium (ranging from 11 to 19), and high (20 and above).

- A sweet potato has 36 grams of carbohydrates, but only 15 grams (3 ¾ teaspoons) of sugar. If you eat this food with butter and a protein, there will be no spike in glucose.

- Ensure Plus has a high GL of 22 and 50 grams of carbohydrates. Those carbohydrates are all in the form of sugar. The Nutrition Facts Label on Ensure Plus says it only has 22 grams (5 ½ teaspoons) of sugar, because maltodextrin is not required to be included in the sugar content on the Nutrition Facts Label. There is a lot of sugar in Ensure, and it has a high GL. Maltodextrin has a GI of 107 which is very high, higher than sugar. (See page 47 for more information on Ensure.)

- Agave Nectar is a sweetener that is being promoted as a healthy food. It is also called the century plant and grows in southwestern United States. I do not consider it a healthy food. The reason the GI and GL are low is because Agave Nectar is 90 percent fructose and only 10 percent glucose. Again, the GI and the GL are solely based on the glucose in a product. Turn to page 60 and find out that the fructose molecule in sugar is a bigger problem than the glucose molecule. Way bigger. Also, Agave Nectar has more concentrated sugar than sugar itself. Do not eat, drink, or put this in your mouth!

- Having a low GI does not necessarily make something a healthy food. Ice cream, for example, falls into the mid range for GI and the low range for GL. The reason for this is because ice cream has fat and protein (which have low GI and GLs and stabilize the sugar) in it, but ice cream can suppress the immune system.

I think the most important factor to look at when you eat a carbohydrate is the sugar content. If your food has a Nutrition Facts Label, you can easily find this out. If not, there are other ways to find this information. See the Resources section on page 141 for more information. If you find there are more than 8 grams (2 teaspoons) of sugar in a food, you should only eat half the portion size in one sitting. You could also pick another food, maybe a food that does not need a label, such as a whole food.

If you'd like to know more about the GI and GL, see the Resources section on page 141. Some of the websites listed there are the ones I used to get my information for this chapter.

ORAL GLUCOSE TOLERANCE TEST AND ALTERNATIVES

By this time, I'm sure you've picked up on my absolute abhorrence of added sugar. So, here's a question: small doses of sugar for diagnostic purposes are perfectly okay, if it means your doctor will be able to tell if you have diabetes, hyperglycemia, or hypoglycemia, right? The short answer is NO!

The oral glucose tolerance test (OGTT) should not be given unless no other test clarifies your situation. Here is the protocol for the test: fast for twelve hours and then take 75 grams (about 19 teaspoons) of glucose in water. The doctor will then test your blood every half-hour for four to six hours. The doctor should also ask how you feel.

The point of the test is to measure how sugar affects the body over time. If blood glucose levels spike or remain elevated throughout the test period, then the diagnosis would be diabetes or hyperglycemia, depending on the severity of the elevated levels. If blood glucose drops below normal, then the diagnosis would be hypoglycemia.

To my knowledge, no researcher has tested for minerals, cholesterol, triglycerides, or white blood cell counts while conducting the OGTT. Since it is my position that these factors help determine health or sickness, I wonder if the researchers would have been unpleasantly surprised had they looked into these factors and found them out of the normal range. Then they would have had to deal with more problems than just the OGTT. Since the body works in harmony, I am sure there is more than one factor out of the normal range when the OGTT is not in the normal range, but it is amazing how the body will come back to homeostasis when sugar is taken out.

Aside from this, the OGTT has many other problems associated with it.

Problems With the Test

Doctors usually administer an OGTT when a patient doesn't feel well and reports symptoms similar to those a diabetic or pre-diabetic would experience. Thus, it is a safe bet that the patient would feel even worse during the test. People who already feel sick will feel worse if there is any kind of sugar assault on their body.

Research has linked myocardial ischemia, a heart disorder caused by insufficient blood flow to heart muscles, to the OGTT. One study used healthy older women, who didn't have high blood pressure or heart disease, as subjects. The subjects did not get enough oxygen in the blood to keep a strong blood flow to the heart during the OGTT—but I feel similar results would be gained by studying any group of people.[1]

Another problem with the OGTT is that the test does not always provide reproducible results. One study of 212 Chinese men and women showed that doctors who gave the OGTT to the same patient twice in one week could only reproduce their results 65.5 percent of the time.[2]

Also, the test doesn't account for allergic reactions to the various types of sugar that contribute to the overall blood glucose level. Some people may be more sensitive to corn, sugarcane, or beets. If the sugar used for the test is derived from only one source, it can skew the results if the patient has an allergy. Corn-based glucose will spike the test if the patient is allergic to corn, but at the same time the test would show little reaction from the other sources of glucose.[3]

Many patients endure some interesting side effects during and after the OGTT. These can include dizziness, vomiting, stomachaches, lightheadedness, or severe headaches. Some patients I talk to say they never felt the same after an OGTT.[4]

There Are Other Options

There are several non-invasive tests for diabetes, metabolic syndrome, and other sugar-related ailments that should be employed before going to the OGTT. First, there is the fasting plasma glucose test. For this test, the patient must fast for twelve hours and then have blood drawn. If the blood glucose level is 99 mg/dL (milligrams of sugar per deciliter of blood) or below, the patient is diagnosed normal. (A deciliter is equal to one-tenth of a liter.) A pre-diabetic would have a range of 100 to 125 mg/dL and a diabetic would spike at 126 mg/dL or above. This test is not always accurate, since some people with a normal fasting blood glucose level fail.[5] Patients can have a normal fasting level, but it could spike later and not be recognized by the fasting test. If this test is used with others, it is a stronger indicator.

Doctors may also call for a glycated hemoglobin test, also known as an A1C test. This test tracks average blood glucose control for two to three months prior to the test. The test itself shows what happens in the body over a three-month time frame. In healthy people, approximately 5 percent of hemoglobin is glycated. Glycated hemoglobin is blood that binds sugar with protein in an abnormal way and causes problems in the body. Diabetics will have higher amounts of glycated hemoglobin. Doctors started using this test as a management tool for diabetics, but now some have recognized the value of this test as a diagnostic tool.[6]

Other doctors may suggest an insulin blood test. Insulin regulates sugar absorption into various cells, including fat cells. High blood glucose levels (like those found after eating) stimulate insulin release. Low blood glucose inhibits insulin levels. This test, when taken after fasting, can diagnose diabetes because high insulin levels during fasting may mean that the pancreas is working too hard, since it is releasing insulin when the body doesn't need it. A doctor will tell the patient whether or not to fast before taking this test.

There are also urine glucose tests to tell whether or not glucose is present in your urine. A paper dipstick is saturated with glucose-sensitive chemicals and dipped into urine. The body doesn't normally excrete glucose in urine unless the glucose levels in the blood are very high. Therefore, if a person's urine has traces of glucose in it, he or she likely has a high blood glucose level, indicating diabetes.

Researchers are also investigating whether certain exhaled gases are markers for diabetes, which would allow for the eventual employment of a breathalyzer-style test patients can blow into. The researchers are studying methyl nitrates, gases that a healthy person expels, and have found that these gases spike in diabetics when they are in a hyperglycemic state. Eventually, there will be a breath test.[7]

Finally, there are always the home blood glucose testing devices (glucometers) available from just about any drugstore in the country. You prick your finger or your arm with a little lance and take a reading. Or, you can fast for twelve hours, take a reading, and then eat a typical meal for you. Prick your finger or arm an hour after eating the meal and compare the results. If the results aren't normal (the manufacturer of the glucometer should provide numbers for a normal range) then I would say that you should immediately start following Food Plan III (see page 112). After following the plan for a week, take a reading again to see if you're making progress. If you aren't, you need to consult with your healthcare provider.

Any of these tests will help you learn more about your body so you can make a determination about your glucose tolerance without having to resort to the OGTT. However, there are always exceptions to the rule. If no other test tells you definitively that you are diabetic, insulin resistant, or hypoglycemic, then you might have to take the OGTT. It will give you the information that you need.

Let me say one more thing. If you or your healthcare provider feel you have a blood sugar problem, do me a favor and go on Food Plan III for two weeks before you have any test, and use the Body Monitor Kit to test for food allergies. Many people just need to stop abusing themselves and their bodies will respond. So, first things first.

CONCLUSION

This is a chapter that you can refer to many times for information to help you choose carbohydrates wisely. The two most important things to remember when choosing wisely are to eat whole foods and choose the carbohydrates that have the least amount of sugar.

Speaking about sugar, the next chapter has lots of sugar in it. In fact, it is oozing with sugar. So leave your spoon in the drawer until after you read all the shocking information—because once you're done reading, you won't want all that food with added sugar.

5

Sugar and the Food We Eat

This chapter is about foods and beverages we put in our mouths that our bodies do not like. Our heads say, "Gimmie, gimmie," and bodies say, "I do not need this!" Many times our heads get their way, getting in the way of our bodies getting and feeling well.

First on the list of bad things we put in our mouths are soft drinks, which give many of us way too many calories. You will find out that these beverages (that are essentially nothing but sugar and chemicals) unfortunately give us a lot more things our bodies don't need besides calories.

Ensure is also a beverage with lots of calories. Some people use Ensure as a meal substitute. This beverage's advertisement says that it is a healthy drink with vitamins and minerals. The manufacturer forgot to tell us that there is so much sugar in the product that it upsets the body chemistry and loses its nutritional value. You will also find out about a product the makers of Ensure produce that is not even required to say how much sugar is in the product on the Nutrition Facts Label.

We add sugar to many processed foods, even though many of them are already sweet. Not only have we forgotten how the original foods taste, but we have made the end result unhealthy. This chapter will teach you how to find out how much natural sugar is in a product and how much sugar is added.

Corn is something that started out as a healthy product, but humans turned much of it into corn syrup that our bodies have a hard time processing. I personally think corn syrup would make a better fuel for cars than it does a sweetener for food.

Chocolate has antioxidants in it, and therefore, it is a healthy food in its raw, unprocessed form. Unfortunately, when the chocolate has been processed it loses some of its nutrients. Then, when sugar is added, the body cannot use the healthy antioxidants present in raw chocolate.

This chapter also includes information on AGEs, unhealthy substances that our bodies make when we eat sugar all the time and our bloodstreams do not have time to process the sugar into the cells or liver.

Read on to get the particulars on these sugary items.

THE HARD FACTS ABOUT SOFT DRINKS

Whether you call it a soft drink, pop, soda, soda pop, or a carbonated drink, this beverage has a lot of added sugar. In fact, it is all added sugar. (See page 56 for more on added sugars.) If it is made with sugar (and isn't sugar-free) and it is 12 ounces (which most soft drinks are), chances are you are getting about 10 teaspoons of sugar per serving. There are other non-alcoholic drinks that have a lot of sugar, also. This section will explain what is in these drinks and how they affect the body.

An Overwhelming Amount

As of 2005, the average American drank 35.5 gallons of regular soft drinks (with sugar, as opposed to diet) and 8.2 gallons of fruit juice per year.[1] (For the record, the term "soft drinks" refers to soda only. The other sugar-laden drinks I discuss are part of a different category.) Twelve ounces of apple, grape, or orange juice (fresh squeezed, canned, or frozen) has the same amount of sugar as a 12-ounce can of soda. There are 128 fluid ounces in a gallon. Let's see, that's 43.7 gallons of drinks. This works out to approximately 466 12-ounce servings of regular soda and fruit juice per person per year. That is close to $1\frac{1}{4}$ 12-ounce cans a day. Of those 466 soda and fruit juice drinks, 379 of them are regular soft drinks (soda).

Diet soda doesn't have sugar in it per se, but the industry uses artificial sweeteners to help give it that sugary taste. On average, Americans drink 171 cans of diet soda per person per year.[2] So, in total, we drink more than 637 12-ounce cans of soda (regular or diet) or fruit juice per person per year.

There are three other categories of non-alcoholic drinks that contain sugar. The first is fruit drinks, which are different than fruit juice because they are made up of a small amount of fruit juice and lots of sugar. The second is drinks that end in -ade, such as Gatorade or lemonade. The third is non-alcoholic cocktail mixers, such as margarita mix. Americans drink 13.9 gallons of drinks from these categories combined per person per year.[3]

The following will give you an example of sugar amounts in these non-alcoholic drinks. An 8-ounce serving of fruit punch has 30 grams (7$\frac{1}{2}$ teaspoons) of sugar. Gatorade has 14 grams (3$\frac{1}{2}$ teaspoons) of sugar per 8-ounce serving. Jose Cuervo Margarita Mix has 24 grams (6 teaspoons) of sugar per 4-ounce serving. That is more sugar than the amount in 4 ounces of Coca-Cola.

Back to soda. The amount of sugar or high fructose corn syrup in each can of soda varies depending on the brand. Suffice it to say 10 teaspoons of sugar is a nice thumbnail average for the amount of sugar in 12-ounce cans of soda (and fruit juice).

Now, why is soda bad for you? Let's start with the fact that people who drink the average amount of regular soda (379 12-ounce cans per year, as I mentioned earlier) are consuming an additional 3,790 teaspoons of sugar or other sweeteners per person per year.

You shouldn't just take my word that soft drinks will slowly do damage to your body and possibly kill you. In 2004, the American Academy of Pediatrics (AAP) made this policy statement in its journal, *Pediatrics:* "Pediatricians should work to eliminate sweetened drinks in schools." The doctors cited obesity and the replacement of nutrients commonly found in whole foods and milk as the primary reasons for this policy change.[4]

Let's look at some of the facts the AAP used when determining this policy statement that all pediatricians are, in theory, required to follow. For each additional serving of soda a child consumes, both body mass index (BMI) and risk of obesity increase (after factors like lifestyle, location, and diet are taken into consideration).[5] These increases were thought to be caused by ingesting sugar energy in liquid form (soft drinks, fruit juice, and other non-alcoholic drinks).[6]

Perhaps it would help if I simplified the concept. An average serving of soda is about 150 calories. Let's say the average child is supposed to consume 2,000 calories per day to maintain a healthy weight and lifestyle. Each soda the child consumes that makes his or her total daily calorie intake greater than 2,000 is associated with weight gain. So, if a child consumes one soda per day, at an average of 150 additional calories per soda, by the end of a year the child will be 15 pounds heavier.

Are You Overweight? Find Out!

A person's BMI measures body fat by taking height and weight into consideration. Although it doesn't actually measure the exact percentage of body fat in an individual, it is a useful tool for determining a healthy average weight for a specific height. Many doctors and nutritionists use the BMI calculation because it provides a simple number that tells patients if they are underweight, normal weight, overweight, or obese, allowing healthcare professionals to discuss any issues that may exist with the patient.

Calculate Your BMI!

Want to know where you'd fall on the BMI scale? Put your height and weight into the equation to see how you measure up.

$$\frac{\text{Weight (in pounds)} \times 703}{\text{Height (in inches)}^2} = \text{BMI}$$

What does your BMI mean? If it's:

- Below 18.5: you are considered underweight.
- Between 18.5 and 24.9: you are considered normal weight.
- Between 25 and 29.9: you are considered overweight.
- Above 30: you are considered obese.

Or, if you'd like the work done for you, head over to the National Heart, Lung, and Blood Institute's website and they'll figure it out. (To find out how to get to the website, see Resources on page 145.)

Even Without Sugar, They're Still Not Good

If the extra sugar in soft drinks isn't enough to make you stop drinking soda and juice, perhaps it is time to go deeper into the ingredient list of the average soft drink to see what else can kill you. Soda ingredients are typically carbonated water (water with carbon dioxide), sweetener, phosphoric acid, artificial and natural flavorings, lactic acid, caffeine, and preservatives. Let's simplify this to carbonated water, sweetener, and chemicals.

After sugar and sweeteners, phosphoric acid is the biggest culprit, which is why it's not even safe to just drink diet soft drinks. Soft drink manufacturers add this chemical so they can keep the carbon in the carbonated water until popping the top of the can releases the gas. Science tells us that taking in phosphoric acid introduces phosphorus into the bloodstream.

Didn't I just mention the calcium-phosphorus ratio? No? Good, you're paying attention. When people eat sugar, usually their phosphorous level drops and their calcium level goes up, but these minerals only work according to a set ratio that never changes. We've discussed how minerals only work in relation to each other, and this is a prime example of that. More calcium and less phosphorous means lots of calcium is sitting around doing nothing. The body doesn't accept idle minerals and treats them like toxins. Various plaques that affect teeth, joints, eyes, and blood vessels are usually primarily composed of non-functioning calcium.

It would seem logical to add phosphorous to counteract the results of sugar consumption. For example, it may seem like drinking a can of soda to get your phosphorous levels back up isn't such a bad idea. But, negative health effects come from having too much phosphorous in the bloodstream as well. If you think powering down a can of soda will counteract that piece of chocolate cake you just ate, remember that you're taking the phosphorous with sugar, caffeine, and other chemicals in the soda that all work in separate ways to suppress the immune system and make you sick.

Phosphoric acid is one scary chemical. It raises phosphorous levels and changes the pH (the acid-alkaline balance) of the body so that it is highly acidic, which is another stress on the body. Phosphoric acid on your internal structures is a serious injury, just as battery acid splashed on your skin would be. Most immune systems would go on strike in a highly acidic environment, another surefire way to get sick.

Many sodas also contain 2-acetyl-4-tetrahydroxybutylimidazole, a mouthful better abbreviated as THI. This is the chemical that gives cola-type sodas their caramel color. THI suppresses the immune system all by itself. This is probably because the digestive system cannot make THI into a substance the body can use. Therefore, the immune system comes to the body's defense to help get the THI out of the body. In fact, Australian researchers recommended that THI be used to treat autoimmune diseases, such as arthritis or lupus, which occur when the immune system overreacts. When the immune system overreacts, it becomes hyperactive. THI suppresses the immune system, or slows it down. The intent is to get the immune system to work properly. It seems more logical to deal with why you have lupus or arthritis rather than to take THI. Suppressing the immune system leads to other problems, like an increased susceptibility to diseases.

The researchers also suggested that THI be used in transplant surgery to prevent organ rejections.[7] In transplant surgery, the immune system overreacts. It wants to get rid of the foreign invader (the organ being transplanted). THI suppresses the immune system, hopefully allowing the transplant to thrive in the body.

Those researchers help make my case for me, since most people do not want their immune system suppressed.

The Other Uses of Soft Drinks

Phosphoric acid is also the main reason why soft drinks have plenty of other rumored uses besides their main role as beverages—uses that can make even an avid soft drink consumer cringe upon hearing them. Coca-Cola is alleged to be an excellent industrial cleaner, having been used successfully to clean both grease and hard mineral stains from toilets and engine parts.

Hey, soft drink consumers, you're drinking an industrial solvent. Do you feel safe now?

Another rumor about soft drinks is their use in India as pesticides. *The Guardian,* one of the best newspapers in London, reported that farmers were using different types of soft drinks to kill bugs instead of more expensive pesticides. The article was fairly short and didn't explain which ingredients in the drinks killed the insects. I think phosphoric acid might do the trick nicely.

The Bottom Line

Most of this data against soft drinks refer to sugar-filled drinks, but sugar-free drinks, especially those with aspartame (better known as NutraSweet, an artificial sweetener), can have their own negative effects. Researchers typically throw sugar-free drinks into the mix as an afterthought and find that some similar changes in body chemistry occur, and the liver takes more of a beating.[8] Aspartame is not a natural food, so the liver has to try to make it into a substance that the body can either metabolize or remove.

I can't stress it enough—stop drinking soda, soft drinks, sports drinks, fruit juice, fruit drinks, cocktail mixes, and drinks ending in -ade! Instead, eat whole fruit for that sugary flavor.

Soft drinks are a primary source of sugar and therefore represent a serious problem in terms of addiction. If your sugar problem is primarily soft drinks or sugar addiction, Food Addicts Anonymous and Food Addicts in Recovery Anonymous can help. (See Resources, page 143.)

ENSURE IS ANYTHING BUT A SURE THING

Sucrose. Corn syrup. Maltodextrin. All are forms of sugar, and all can be found on the ingredient list for Ensure, a "healthy" drink made by Abbott Laboratories. Ensure is given to elderly people when they cannot consume whole food as they recover from an operation or sickness. Some people use them not only as meal substitutes, but also as a between-meal drink to add calories. Meal substitutes scare me to the point where I wonder if the Food and Drug Administration (FDA) or the Federal Trade Commission (FTC) will ever pull them from the market for deceptive advertising. If you're wondering why I feel this way, read on to learn more about Ensure.

The Label Will Deceive You

Did I mention that manufacturers sometimes break up the sugar in their products by spreading it among many forms of sweetener on the ingredients label, making it seem like the total amount of sugar is less than it really is? For example, the top four ingredients listed for Ensure are water, sugar (sucrose), corn syrup, and maltodextrin (a refined cornstarch). For Ensure, it seems like the primary ingredient is water because water is listed first. However, sucrose, corn syrup, and maltodextrin (all forms of sugar) are listed consecutively in the next three slots. There is a lot of sugar in this product.

Regular Ensure has 40 grams (10 teaspoons) of total carbohydrates per 8-ounce bottle. The company also makes a drink called Ensure Plus, which has 50 grams (12 $1/2$ teaspoons) per bottle. It is confusing because the label for regular Ensure says there are only 22 grams of sugar (sucrose) per bottle. The other 18 grams come from maltodextrin. (Details about maltodextrin will be presented in the following section.) Therefore, all the grams of carbohydrates in Ensure and Ensure Plus come from sugar. Coca-Cola also has 40 grams of sugar per 12-ounce can. So, let's get this straight: the "healthy" liquid meal substitute and the unhealthy soda have exactly the same amount of sugar, but the "healthy" drink delivers this sugar in a solution that is one-third more concentrated? In other words, if you drink equal amounts of Ensure and Coca-Cola, Ensure would give you $1^1/_2$ times the amount of sugar. What comedian tagged this product with the word "healthy"? Even if you just consider the sucrose content of Ensure, that's still 5$\frac{1}{2}$ teaspoons per bottle, which is a lot for one 8-ounce drink. How can a drink that can basically be called sweetened water be considered a healthy meal substitute?

Ensure also contains vitamins and minerals, which is probably why the label claims the drink is "complete, balanced nutrition to help stay healthy, active, and energetic." This is a concern for me because I see older people buying this product at the supermarket all the time. They fill their carts with Ensure, all the while not knowing how unhealthy it really is for them.

The Big Four

Let's go back to the top four ingredients in Ensure for a moment to show why "healthy" and "active" may be oxymorons on this label:

- *Water.* I can't fault water—though for the most part, we live in civilized places where water is piped right into our houses and may need only a little filtration to be healthy. It's almost as if when we buy products with water in them, we are being charged a rate well above what we pay for our tap and filtration.

- *Sugar.* As this book will teach you, sugar does horrible things to your body, largely because it is acidic and forces the body to leech minerals out of the bloodstream to buffer against the acidity. Once these minerals have been removed, the mineral relationships change and eventually suppress the immune system, leading to diabetes, cancer, metabolic syndrome, and a myriad of other diseases that will be discussed later in the book. (See Chapter 6, page 71.)

- *Corn syrup.* Corn syrup has been linked to many of the same ailments as sugar, such as diabetes, heart disease, and cancer. However, the many different blends of corn syrup are collectively linked to obesity at greater rates than regular sugar. This is because of the high fructose content, which is broken down in the liver and turned directly into fat. Soft drinks also use corn syrup (sometimes called high fructose corn syrup) and are thus highly associated with obesity.

- *Maltodextrin.* Maltodextrin is a carbohydrate that is usually made from refined cornstarch, but can also be made from corn or rice. It

is very high on the glycemic index (GI), with a GI of 100, largely because it breaks down very rapidly. GI measures the rate at which an individual food raises blood sugar levels. Any food with a GI of 55 or lower is considered to be in the low GI range. When the blood sugar level rises for any reason, insulin has to be secreted to bring the blood sugar back to homeostasis. This means there is a fast and high insulin response in maltodextrin since it has a GI of 100. Many times when I read about maltodextrin on the Web, the information tells people to check with their doctors before eating it if they are diabetic. To me, that is a red flag. Whether people are diabetic or not, they should think seriously before they eat or drink much maltodextrin. Some serious athletes like to drink sport drinks and other drinks with maltodextrin in them because they raise the blood sugar fast and high and can provide a surge of energy. For the rest of us, it is better not to have drinks with mal-todextrin because we do not need that spike in blood sugar which can, over time, be a problem. Maltodextrin is also used as a filler. A filler is a cheap food that food companies mix with whatever their product is in order to make boxes, cartons, or cans of the product appear more full. This way, the companies don't have to use expensive foods. Maltodextrin is also used as a food preser-vative. If that sounds like it might be good, it's not. The less sugar and preservatives we put into our bodies, the better off we are.

Regardless of which sweetener is listed first, they all unbalance your body chemistry. My position is that supplemental vitamins and minerals (like the ones in Ensure) are useless when taken with sugar. However, many doctors don't accept this premise, which explains how Ensure and various brands with similar ingredients can label themselves as "healthy." The thinking is that these drinks have vita-mins and minerals in them and that the sugar content has no affect on how these vitamins and minerals are absorbed. Thus, the drinks are considered healthy—until opinion changes and sugar's affect on body chemistry becomes more accepted. Oooh! That thought makes me tingle, but it hasn't happened yet.

To put these liquid meal replacements into context, you need to understand you'd do just as well washing down a multivitamin with soda. In terms of health, this is not a good thing. But in terms of finances, this is a Godsend. Ensure sells for around $5 for 32 ounces. The same amount of soda sells for about $1. You'd just have to factor in the cost of the multivitamin (which varies), and you've got yourself a meal substitute. Many fast food places have all-you-can-drink soda bars, so there are ways to make the unit cost of your sugar death very cheap indeed. At least regular soda doesn't label itself as healthy.

PediaSure—Ensure for Babies

Abbott Laboratories also makes a product for babies and children called PediaSure. Most anxious to find out how much sugar was in a bottle, I went to PediaSure's website. The most information I found there was that PediaSure is "Complete Balanced Nutrition

Another Meal Substitute:
Intravenous Feeding

As I mentioned, Ensure is also used as a meal substitute for elderly people while they are recovering from an operation or illness. That brings me to another subject that is dear to my heart—intravenous feeding (IV), also called total parenteral nutrition. Patients get this at a hospital or in their homes. When a person's digestive system is not ready to resume its work after an operation or illness, he or she is put on an IV—usually for a day or two, but sometimes for a week or more. This meal substitute is a mixture of sugar water, amino acids, vitamins, minerals, other supplements, and sometimes fatty acids and pharmaceutical drugs. It is the only means of nourishment until the patient's digestive system is ready to work again.

The reason sugar is added to the IVs is for calories, but most people can go a few days without calories. A diabetic gets an IV without the sugar, so why can't everyone else?

When we are sick, we have upset body chemistry. Our body needs all the help it can get to heal from an operation or sickness. It does not need sugar suppressing the immune system. The immune system needs to work for us—not against us.

If you need an operation, begin discussing a no-sugar IV during the planning stages, not just right before the operation. I am sure you will have happier endings from the operation or sickness without sugar. To get an IV without sugar, all a patient needs to do is ask his or her anesthesiologist.

for Children's Health." The company listed the ingredients on the website, including the amount of carbohydrates in the drink—but not the amount of sugar. So, I went to a store and looked at a bottle. Sure enough, it was the same thing. No amount of sugar was given. (See Figure 5.1)

I don't give up easily, so I phoned the company's 800 number and talked to a customer service representative. I asked her why the sugar content was not listed on the bottles or on PediaSure's website. I was told that PediaSure falls under the classification of medicine, and therefore does not have to show the sugar content. It does show everything else that is in the product on the Nutritional Facts Label, which is on the back of human-made food products. But, the nice sales representative did tell me how much sugar is in PediaSure: every 8-ounce bottle of the chocolate flavor has 31 grams of carbohydrates (24 of them are sucrose, which equals 6 teaspoons of sugar). Why does a baby have to have chocolate? Why can't we feed our babies baby food and watered-down juice (3/4 pure water and 1/4 apple, orange, or grape juice)? The other 7 grams of carbohydrates in the drink come from maltodextrin. "The only product we consider as sugar is sucrose," I was told. That would mean that even without the maltodextrin, there are 24 grams of sugar in PediaSure, a drink for children and babies. That's more sugar than Ensure contains. Why must we get our babies started on sugar and chocolate so early in life?

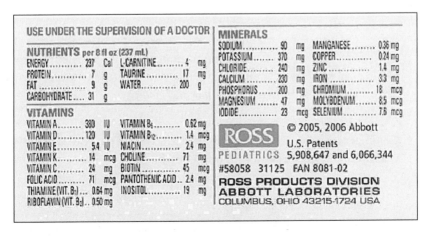

FIGURE 5.1 PEDIASURE LABEL.

Substitutes for Sugar-Laden Liquid Meals

We have already established that meal substitutes aren't very healthy. However, there are some people out there saying, "Great! But I still have problems with solid foods, and I need more calories. What now?" Therefore, I've come up with some suggestions of foods you can prepare as a substitute for Ensure or other sugar-laden drinks.

• Try different brands of baby food. Beech-Nut is a company that doesn't have any added sugar or salt in its products. Baby food is easy to eat, and if you need to gain weight, choose the foods with the most calories. Check out other baby foods for a variety in diet. Both adults and children who have problems digesting food or need more calories can benefit from baby food. (For more on Beech-Nut, see Resources, page 142.)

• Purée fruits. You can purée a lot at a time and they will last about three days in your refrigerator. If you are prediabetic, diabetic, hypoglycemic, have cancer, or have a yeast infection, I do not recommend that you eat fruit until you have your condition under control. There is too much sugar in fruit.

• Cook and then purée vegetables. If you want to use frozen vegetables for convenience sake, do it. Add some butter and a little salt and mix the vegetables together to get a variety of tastes. Remember, herbs and spices help to excite the taste pallet. Again, these will last for about three days.

• Look through the canned and frozen sections of your grocery store. Different stores have different items. Canned puréed pumpkin is almost always there. I have also found puréed squash and other vegetables. However, you should use frozen fruits and vegetables over canned ones whenever possible.

• Cook ground beef, turkey, chicken, or lamb as you normally would and purée it with puréed vegetables.

• Cook and mash potatoes or sweet potatoes. Add butter. For a different flavor, mix them together.

A final point to remember is to accept **no** substitutes for real food!

Your Goose is Overcooked

In 1912, a Frenchman by the name of Louis Maillard found out that the reason some foods discolor and toughen when they cook is due to a chemical attachment between the glucose in the food and the protein in the food. This reaction was deemed the Maillard reaction. Maillard called the product that is formed by the Maillard reaction glycated protein, or Advanced Glycated End Products (AGEs).

The Maillard Reaction Forms AGEs

The Maillard reaction causes toast to turn brown and steak to toughen during cooking. It uses high temperatures to bind the glucose and protein molecules. Maillard found out that this attachment changed the structure of the protein, and that it could be a problem for this new structure of food to digest, assimilate, and metabolize in the body.

Besides barbecuing and frying, when foods are processed by manufacturers, many are heated at high temperatures. Heating food at temperatures over 245°F causes a very rapid increase in AGEs, indicated by the browning of the product. These foods can have intense, tasty flavors people like to eat. Many food manufacturers have taken advantage of this fact, greatly increasing the amount of AGEs in processed food over the last fifty years and sometimes even adding synthetic AGEs.[9]

Sugar and AGEs

Research has shown that this same reaction (sugar binding with protein in an abnormal way) can occur in the body when our blood glucose becomes, and stays, elevated. This reaction has nothing to do with heating or browning.

As I have said, people on average eat over 140 pounds of sugar per person per year.[10] This glut of sugar can cause some people to have continually elevated blood glucose—many more people than in the past, when we ate less sugar. When we eat sugar all day long, our blood sugar never has a chance to come back to homeostasis, or if it does, it doesn't stay there for long. When our blood and our blood cells become awash with sugar continually, the sugar can bind nonenzymatically with protein.

That might not sound so harmful, but it is. There is a normal process where sugar binds enzymatically with protein in our body to form glycoproteins (sugar proteins) that are essential to the working of our body. All of these chemical reactions in living tissues are under strict enzymatic control and conform to a tightly regulated metabolic program. When enzymes attach glucose to proteins, they do so at a specific site, on a specific molecule, for a specific purpose. For instance, these glyco- proteins help strengthen the cell wall, which is constructed out of pro- tein. The body turns normal glycoproteins into enzymes, muscle tissue, tendons, and all the other muscle structures necessary for life. Some of the enzymes created govern the formation of glycoproteins, so we loop back to the beginning of the cycle. They are also used as protective agents and lubricants in the blood.

Sugar and protein are not supposed to bind nonenzymatically. When they do, the products that form are the same as the products formed from browning protein at a high temperature—AGEs. This process can permanently alter the molecular structure of the protein and, as a result, alter the way the AGEs function in the body. The protein becomes toxic to the body.

AGEs and Disease

Since the body does not like toxicity, it calls on the immune system to come to the rescue and remove the toxic substances. Over time, this exhausts the immune system and degeneration slowly sets in. These changes can start as minor disturbances or disabilities, such as allergies, high blood pressure, or headaches, and can later continue on to become specific illnesses, such as heart disease, cancer, or diabetes.

AGEs are characterized as having brown or fluorescent pigments and seem to be linked to many age-related complications, such as athero- sclerosis (the hardening of plaque on the artery walls), hypertension, mac- ular degeneration (a loss of vision in the center of the eye that can lead to blindness), joint stiffness, rheumatoid arthritis, Alzheimer's disease, cataracts, and diabetes.[11,12,13,14,15]

A study presented at the annual meeting of the American Diabetes Association in San Francisco shows that eating browned foods may also cause heart attacks, strokes, and nerve damage.

Scientists have known for many years that cooking proteins with sug- ars in the absence of water can form AGEs that can damage tissues in the body. Cooking with water prevents sugars from binding to proteins to form these poisonous chemicals.

Diabetics suffer a very high incidence of nerve, artery, and kidney damage because high blood sugar levels in their bodies markedly accelerate the chemical reactions that form AGEs.[16]

Some research shows that vegetarians can accumulate more AGEs than meat eaters. They do not get the protein from meat, but they do eat lots of fruit. The higher the sugar content in fruits, the more AGEs vegetarians can accumulate.[17]

Tobacco smoke is another well-documented source of AGEs. Sugar is a commonly added ingredient to tobacco in the United States. This is in addition to the small amount of sugar the tobacco leaf already contains. So, is it the sugar that causes the AGEs, the tobacco smoke, or both?

Since tobacco smoke is absorbed through the lungs, it adds to the body's load of AGEs and creates higher risks of heart attacks, cancer, and other diseases smoking is known to cause.[18]

How to Slow AGEs Down

Cooking without water causes sugars to combine with proteins to form AGEs. So in a perfect world, baking, roasting, and broiling, which can cause AGEs, would be severely limited, while boiling and steaming would be encouraged. According to these findings, brown foods, such as cookies, bread crust, basted meats, and even coffee beans may increase nerve damage, particularly in diabetics who are unusually susceptible to it.

Attempts to modify the progression of diseases linked to AGEs by using drug treatment have had little success on humans.[19] Personally, I think it's crazy for the scientific community to look for a pill to give someone who has eaten over-processed foods or too much sugar simply to stop the Maillard reaction. Who knows what kind of side effects this pill may have?[20]

Food scientists are continually trying to find a method to slow or stop the Malliard reaction in processed food. But, the best way to stop the Maillard reaction is to minimize your intake of processed food and sugar. Once you've weaned yourself from sugar, I guarantee there will be no side effects if you do this.

On the other hand, since steamed vegetables, whole grains, and beans are cooked with water, they do not contain significant amounts of AGEs. This is certainly another reason to remove as much sugar as possible from your diet as soon as possible, and to eat much of your food raw or steamed.

This is where the barbecue master standing at the grill may argue that man has been roasting and browning food over an open flame since the discovery of fire, long before AGEs became a cause for concern. Others may rightly point out that archaeological records date the emergence of diseases linked to the Maillard reaction to long after man started roasting food. Both of these statements are correct. In fact, the emergence of said diseases coincides with a different (although not surprising) event in history—the introduction of sugar into the modern diet.

MORE THAN A SPOONFUL OF SUGAR
IN PROCESSED FOODS

Every processed food has a Nutrition Facts Label. Now that you know that 4 grams equals 1 teaspoon, you can tell that there are 11 teaspoons of sugar in the apple yogurt, Figure 5.2 (page 57). But, you cannot tell how much sugar is in the yogurt, how much is in the apples, or how much is added sugar.

Added sugars are defined as those sugars added to foods and beverages during processing or home preparation. Until 2006, this information was difficult to get and it is still not easy to get for specific items. Hopefully in the future the manufacturer will be required to put this information on the Nutrition Facts Label.

Every food label also has to have the ingredients listed. You can see from the following ingredient list that there is high fructose corn syrup in the apple yogurt, but you still do not know how much.

INGREDIENTS: CULTURED GRADE A REDUCED FAT MILK, APPLES, HIGH FRUCTOSE CORN SYRUP, CINNAMON, NUTMEG, NATURAL FLAVORS, AND PECTIN. CONTAINS ACTIVE YOGURT AND ACIDOPHILUS CULTURES.

How Much of the Sugar You Eat Is Naturally Occurring?

There is no line for added sugar on a product's Nutrition Facts Label. The sugar amount you see on the label is the total sugar in the product.

Nutrition Facts

Serving Size 1 container (227g)

Amount Per Serving

Calories 240	Calories from Fat 25

	% Daily Value*
Total Fat 3g	4%
Saturated Fat 1.5g	9%
Trans Fat 0g	
Cholesterol 15mg	5%
Sodium 140mg	6%
Total Carbohydrate 46g	15%
Dietary Fiber Less than 1g	3%
Sugars 44g	
Protein 9g	

Vitamin A	2%	•	Vitamin C	4%
Calcium	35%	•	Iron	0%

*Percent Daily Values are based on a 2,000 calorie diet. Your daily values may be higher or lower depending on your calorie needs.

FIGURE 5.2
NUTRITION FACTS
LABEL FOR
APPLE YOGURT.

This can be deceiving and confusing. The reader has no idea how much sugar occurs naturally in a product and how much has been added by the manufacturer.

In the United States, the average person consumes about 74 pounds of added sugar per year, according to survey data from 1999 to 2002. The data were analyzed by researchers at the Beltsville Human Nutrition Research Center's Community Nutrition Research Group. That's about 23 teaspoons of added sugar every day—460 calories that supply no additional nutrients and upset the body's chemistry. Keep in mind the average person consumes 142 pounds of sugar each year (added and otherwise), so the amount of added sugar taken in by each person is actually more than half the total amount of sugar consumed.

Most of this added sugar goes to the following products: regular soft drinks (with sugar, non-diet), candy, pies, fruit drinks, milk-based desserts and products (ice cream, sweetened yogurt, and sweetened milk), and grain products (cakes and cookies).

How Is Added Sugar Calculated?

There seems to be no analytical method for distinguishing between added sugar and naturally occurring sugar, so the added sugar values are calculated by using the sugars listed as label ingredients and the nutrient values for total sugars and total carbohydrates in the product.[21] This is the method the government used to calculate the added sugar, and it works for most processed foods. Unfortunately, the government did not do any brand-name foods, but you can still get an idea of how much sugar has been added to many products.

There are some minor oddities to how added sugar is calculated. For example, if the product has an artificial sweetener in it, the artificial sweetner is not shown as added sugar. Sugar alcohols, such as mannitol, sorbitol, and xylitol, are not included in added sugars either, although they must be included in the ingredient list.

Sugar alcohols are carbohydrates mostly manufactured from sugars and starches. Part of their chemical structure resembles sugar, and part of it resembles alcohol, but they cannot get you drunk. Because they are not completely absorbed, they can ferment in the intestines and cause bloating, gas, or diarrhea.

The main place sugar alcohols are used is in sugar-free gum. I think manufacturers use them in food because sugar alcohols do not have to be on the Nutrition Facts Label. Sugar alcohols have about one-half the calories as sugar. Since they are not a whole food and have no nutritional value, I see no reason to put them in your mouth.

One more problem is that the government charts measure product values in grams. For the government's purposes, the individual serving size used for the statistics is 100 grams of the food, or about 25 teaspoons (which is equivalent to $1/4$ cup). Note that when a product is advertised as having reduced fat, it often means more sugar has been added to make it tastier.

Table 5.1 lists a few examples to show the incredible amount of sugar that is added to some products. You can find many more examples at the U.S. Department of Agriculture's website (see Resources, page 146).[22]

There are 2,037 different products in the government's tables. Be ready—you can spend days checking this data on their website.

Natural sugars in fruits, vegetables, and other foods provide the products with vitamins and minerals, which are important to the body. Most important of all is the fiber that can be found in whole

TABLE 5.1		ADDED SUGAR VALUES FOR CERTAIN FOODS					
Food	Carbs (grams)	Naturally-Occurring Sugar (grams)	(tsps)	Added Sugar (grams)	(tsps)	Total Sugar (grams)	(tsps)
Cookies, oatmeal, regular*	69	6	1½	19	4¾	25	6¼
Cookies, oatmeal, fat free*	79	15	3¾	27	6¾	42	10½
Beans, baked, canned with pork & sweet sauce	21	1	¼	8	2	9	2¼
Peanut butter, added sugar, smooth style	20	6	1½	3	¾	9	2¼
Peanut butter, smooth style, reduced fat	36	4	1	4	1	8	2
Breakfast bar, corn flake crust with fruit	73	1	¼	34	8½	35	8¾
Croissants, butter	46	1	¼	10	2½	11	2¾
Frozen yogurts, flavors other than chocolate	22	5	1¼	16	4	21	5¼

* Commercially prepared

foods and not in added sugars. The fiber makes the food travel slowly through the digestive system, giving the body what it needs.
Added sugars that are found in refined carbohydrates are digested
quickly and can move into the bloodstream and upset the body
chemistry rapidly. It seems that both the speed of the sugar entering
the bloodstream and the amount of sugar eaten upset body chemistry, throwing the body out of homeostasis.

This information about added sugars is new. I am sure in the
future there will be changes made to the government charts. New
information will emerge, but for now this is the first step to understanding how much added sugar is in many products.

CHOCOLATE GOODNESS???

Hey! Did you hear that chocolate is good for you? Apparently, the
cocoa bean, which is where chocolate comes from, comes loaded
with antioxidants called flavanols. These antioxidants lower cholesterol and blood sugar and open vessels to reduce blood pressure.

Fructose Roulette

As a nation, we're overweight and crashing from a sugar buzz into full-blown type-2 diabetes at never-before-seen rates. In 2005, 20.8 million people (7 percent of the population) had diabetes.[23]

Many nutritionists and other healthcare providers have linked this trend to dietary changes and declining physical activity. As for exercise, you can see with your own eyes that active people are healthier than lazy people. I'm not in the business of chasing you off your couch with a Stun Gun—but perhaps I can provide information on the dietary changes that have gone hand-in-hand with our sloth to bring us to this state. For the most part, it can be summed up with one scary word: fructose.

Depending on which dictionary you use, the definition of a food is any substance that is or can be consumed by living organisms to sustain life or supply energy or nourishment. I do not think that fructose supplies nourishment, but it does supply calories (energy). Therefore, I have included it in this chapter about sugar and food.

All About Fructose

If you didn't already know, sugar was brought from India to Europe. The European sweet tooth fueled slavery, and then sugar and slavery were brought to the new world. Picking sugar beets and sugarcane is hard work, and therefore, not many people wanted to do it. Slaves had no choice.

The civilized world started its addiction to sugar with sucrose, which is derived from beets and sugarcane. Sucrose is actually a 50/50 blend of glucose and fructose. Glucose and fructose are simple sugars that are metabolized differently in the body. With glucose, when blood sugar levels rise after we eat a meal, the pancreas releases insulin that "mops up" the glucose from the bloodstream and carries it to the cells for energy. Fructose is absorbed in a different way. It is rapidly metabolized by the liver—with complications, as you will soon learn.

In the 1970s, a new player hit town: corn sweetener. The sugar blends in corn syrup (called dextrose, dextrin, fructose, and/or high fructose corn syrup) can be lumped together as a class of chemicals that all have similar effects. Enzymes turn cornstarch into both fructose and glucose, resulting in blends ranging from 42 percent to 80 percent fructose. The remaining percentage is glucose. Soft drink manufacturers typically use the 55 percent fructose blend.

High fructose corn syrup and its cousins have exploded on to the market even more than sucrose has because they are cheaper to produce. These chemicals from corn became the new miracle sweetener. Some doctors said they were okay even for diabetics because fructose does not raise blood sugar levels the way glucose does.[24]

This is nonsense, as you will find out. Needless to say, corn-based fructose is in nearly everything, even replacing glucose in hospital IV bags given to patients.

It wasn't just being a cheaper alternative to sucrose that caused corn-based fructose to pop up everywhere. It also helps food brown better than sucrose does. I have discussed the Maillard reaction (food browning) on page 53, linking it to cancer, diabetes, and other maladies.

All sugars are subject to this reaction, but fructose reacts seven times faster than glucose, resulting in toxic and/or less functional proteins in the body.[25]

Maillard products can slow the metabolism of amino acids and other nutrients, like zinc. This can lead to undigested proteins. The undigested proteins have carcinogenic (cancer-causing) properties. These products have also been linked to signs of aging and clinical complications of diabetes, such as eye diseases and kidney failure.[26]

The Effects of Fructose

Studies indicate that fructose raises the cholesterol and low-density lipoproteins (LDL) in the bloodstream in most subjects, regardless of whether the people had been classified as having healthy or unhealthy blood glucose tolerance.[27]

It is almost a universal belief that elevated cholesterol and LDLs lead to heart disease. Even the very low-density lipoproteins (VLDL) increase in the presence of sugar, which can lead to similar results. This occurs without an apparent change in high-density lipoproteins (HDL).[28]

Most doctors say that VLDL and LDL levels should be low and HDL levels should be as high as possible in a healthy person.

Continuing on with heart disease indicators, fructose has also been shown to raise triglyceride levels in the bloodstream significantly. Triglycerides are the form in which most fat is stored in the body. Early man ate fructose from fresh fruit, but today we eat and drink much more fructose—not only from fruit, but also from soft drinks, candy, desserts, and the like. The liver cannot handle these large amounts of fructose and turns the excess fructose into triglycerides.

In one study, men, young women, and post-menopausal women were given fat-free diets containing calcium and a substance that was either 40 percent fructose and 60 percent starch or 40 percent glucose and 60 percent starch. According to this study, men are susceptible to the triglyceride reaction to fructose, showing a 32 percent increase in triglycerides after eating sugar. The young women in the studies were unaffected, but post-menopausal women also had an increase in triglycerides. Results in a parallel rat study showed similar increases in triglycerides across both genders.[29]

Getting back to fructose absorption (or lack thereof), the fructose that the body doesn't convert to glucose or fat has been linked to quite a few disorders. A study of twenty-five people who had functional bowel disease or irritable bowel syndrome (IBS) showed that even small quantities of improperly absorbed fructose can cause problems.[30]

In a more comprehensive study, 50 percent of women who were classified as not being able to absorb fructose well developed IBS symptoms after eating fructose. IBS is a common disorder of the intestines that leads to cramps, gassiness, bloating, and changes in bowel habits ranging from diarrhea to constipation. The study also tested for PMS and depression, and found increases with these afflictions as well.[31]

Many people with blood test results that show high triglycerides also have a high uric acid count. Uric acid is a product of purines, which are a part of all human tissue and are found in many foods, such as beef, lamb, pork, and yeast. Uric acid increases greatly in solution with a high fructose sweetener. Comparisons to sucrose did not show an elevated uric acid count. Uric acid is widely considered to be an indicator of both gout (uric acid deposits in the joints) and heart disease.[32]

Another acid that seems to increase with fructose as opposed to sucrose is lactic acid. Lactic acid is formed by the fermentation of sugar. People with preexisting acidotic conditions like diabetes, postoperative stress, or uremia (buildup of waste products in the blood due to the kidney's inability to excrete them) are most vulnerable to lactic acid buildups. Ultra-high concentrations of lactic acid cause metabolic acidosis (elevated acid in the blood) which can result in death.[33]

Ingesting too much fructose can also lead to diarrhea.[34] When we eat too much sugar, the pancreas tries to squirt insulin at it and then sends it to the liver to be processed into fatty acids. Whatever sugar can't be dealt with in this way is excreted in urine and feces. Fructose becomes fat in the liver much faster than sucrose or glucose, because the body doesn't readily break it down into glucose unless necessary.[35] This suggests why obesity is exploding in our society. Fructose also causes insulin receptors to lose sensitivity, resulting in more insulin being pumped out to digest glucose.[36]

Both fructose and sucrose have been linked to wrinkles as cellular metabolism breaks down, leading to oxidation damage of the collagen in the skin. In rat studies, fructose raised these markers to a higher degree than sucrose. The research went as far as to say that the similar damage caused by sucrose was caused by the naturally occurring fructose in it, rather than the sucrose itself.[37]

To relate fructose to homeostasis, fructose seems to have an effect on many enzymes and hormones in the body and the mineral relationships that govern the reactions between them. In several different studies, mineral relationships in subjects seemed to be altered. A rat study found that fructose consistently outpaced pure glucose for creation of excess calcium in the kidney, while spiking phosphorous and magnesium levels in the urine. The urine pH was also more acidic with fructose than with glucose.[38]

A study performed on humans showed spiked excretions of other minerals, like iron and magnesium, along with the ones revealed in the rat study.[39]

I have contended that these mineral relationships are the core of proper health. If sugar throws off the body chemistry, no enzyme or hormone will work properly, resulting in illness.

Fructose also causes copper to metabolize poorly. Copper deficiencies have been linked to fragile bones, anemia, defects in connective tissue, infertility, heart arrhythmias, high cholesterol, and spiked blood sugar levels.[40]

On a side note, most of the corn in the United States (where corn sweetener comes from) has been genetically modified (GM). GM means genes have been added, rearranged, or replaced in the product through genetic engineering. If corn has had genes added, rearranged, or replaced, its chemical configuration has been changed. We evolved from early man, who had digestive enzymes to help metabolize foods in certain chemical configurations. If we change the chemical configuration of the food we eat, by GM or over-processing our food, our enzymes will not work as well. This book is not about GM foods, but since almost all corn has been genetically modified, it seems a prudent idea to eat as little corn sweetener as possible because you will get a double whammy—corn syrup and GM food. Both processes, making corn into sweetener and genetically modifying the corn, make the sweetener difficult to digest and metabolize.

Finally, fructose stimulates overeating and obesity. Eating glucose releases insulin and the hormone leptin, which tell the body to stop eating. Eating fructose, however, releases the hormone ghrelin, which tells the body to keep eating because it is hungry.[41]

Between the increased fat production in the liver and the stimulated overeating from ghrelin, is it any wonder that Americans are losing the battle of the waistline? Fructose is a major culprit in a vicious cycle of eating poorly, feeling poorly, and then repeating—not because we desire to but because we are addicted.

What Happens Next?

If you give up added fructose in your diet, you will have to give up glucose as well. Most added sugar has both fructose and glucose in it, such as beet sugar, cane sugar, high fructose corn syrup, honey, and others. It's just that the fructose molecule is a bigger problem than the glucose molecule is. The food plans at the end of this book (see page 112) are all designed to help you live a sugar-free lifestyle.

So stop drinking soda. Replace desserts with whole fruit. You may have to put up with high fructose corn syrup in your ketchup (even the "all-natural" ketchups at health food stores have some), but the amount of fructose in an average splash of ketchup is nothing compared to what is in the average person's soda intake.

With the assertions and citations listed here, perhaps your eyes have been opened to the hazards of excessive fructose ingestion. People who have medical problems are even more sensitive to fructose, but soon enough even healthy people may have problems.

We know this because researchers associated with the Harvard Medical School went to an isolated area of Panama, the San Blas Islands, where the Kuma Indians live. The researchers studied the natives, who drank a cocoa drink made with raw chocolate—but we'll discuss that a little later.[42]

For the record, chocolate company Mars, Inc. paid for this research into the isolated Indian tribe. A little PR placement by Mars, and suddenly the public sees a run on "healthy" dark chocolate. However, what Mars forgot to mention is that commercially available dark chocolate still has tons of sugar in it. In my days as a sugar and chocolate addict, I don't think I was ever brave enough to consume unsweetened cocoa, without fat or sugar. I'm told it is very bitter.

Is Chocolate *Really* Good for You?

I will be the first to admit that in the case of unsweetened chocolate, the antioxidant qualities normally outweigh the risks from the other ingredients. However, that is not the case with processed chocolate. The biggest problem with chocolate is and always has been sugar, which is why I've included a section on chocolate in a book about sugar.

Another problem with chocolate is that the act of processing the cocoa beans—grinding and washing them, etc.—can reduce the antioxidant benefits in the final product being sold to the public. Also, many chocolate blends are alkalized, which reduces acidity and raises the pH.[43] This type of chocolate is darker, milder in taste, and less acidic than non-alkalized cocoa.

Sometimes, it is the fat content of the chocolate mix that lowers the healthy effects of chocolate. In milk chocolate the cocoa is extremely overwhelmed by sugar, and therefore, has less antioxidants than all other types of chocolate (dark, semi-sweet, baking chocolate, etc.).

The Original Recipe

As I mentioned, chocolate's antioxidant qualities were first discovered when Mars paid for researchers to study the ancient Kuma Indian tribe's use of cocoa. The researchers discovered that the natives drank a cocoa drink made with raw chocolate and bitter herbs. The cocoa beans were found to be loaded with antioxidants. In a diet of native food and the absence of sugar, the people were healthy.

The following facts are in the records of the Cortez Expedition from Spain into Mexico to conquer the Aztec Indians. Montezuma, the Aztec emperor, served unsweetened chocolate mixed with Jalapeño peppers and possibly vanilla, herbs, and other spices to the Spanish troops while trying to figure out whether to attack, run, or surrender. Alas, Montezuma lost the battle. After defeating the Aztecs, Cortez brought samples of cocoa back to Spain with him.[44]

Spain may have had the chocolate, but Britain had the sugar. History doesn't tell us who suggested that the cocoa needed a sweetener, but we do know which is more valuable.

Chocolate was never the same after sucrose was added to it. Honey, fructose, or corn syrup would have done similar things to chocolate. A study that specifically left out unsweetened chocolate showed that it didn't matter what the chocolate was sweetened with—the level of triglycerides in the blood of the person who ate it still went up. Triglycerides are a form of fat produced in the liver. The more sugar people consume, the higher the triglycerides.[45]

Just a PR Stunt?

As an example of how sugar makes chocolate a horrible food, let's consider Mars's CocoaVia line of "healthy" chocolate products. Freshly buoyed with research into flavanols, the various products of CocoaVia are touted as having lots of antioxidants for healthy hearts. The line was originally only available on the Internet, but was shipped to retail stores in September 2005. Various vitamins are listed on the Nutrition Facts Label, and they all range between 10 and 25 percent of the Recommended Daily Allowance (RDA). Oh, wow! So in addition to the flavanols there is up to 25 percent RDA of Vitamin C or B12? Sign me up, right? Wrong! Each CocoaVia chocolate bar (there are seven different kinds) is about 22 grams.[46] Twenty-two grams of chocolate is not that much. It is like eating four and one-half Hershey's Kisses. The average candy bar that you get at your grocery or drug store is about 40 grams. A 22-ounce candy bar is considered a snack bar. However, each CocoaVia bar has between 6 and 12 grams (between 1 1/2 and 3 teaspoons) of sugar added to the chocolate. That's a lot of sugar for one small, "healthy" chocolate bar.

The bar with the most sugar is the CocoaVia Milk Chocolate Bar, with 12 grams (3 teaspoons) of sugar, which seems to defeat the very

CocoaVia™ Rich Chocolate Indulgence Beverage Nutrition Facts

Nutrition Facts	Amount/Serving	%DV*	Amount/Serving	%DV*
Serv. Size 1 bottle (5.65 oz.)	Total Fat 3g	5%	Total Carb. 28g	9%
	Sat. Fat 1g	5%	Fiber 3g	12%
	Trans Fat 0g		Sugars 24g	
Calories 150 Fat Cal. 25	Cholest. 5mg	2%	Protein 6g	
	Sodium 135mg	6%		

*Percent Daily Values (DV) are based on a 2,000 calorie diet.

Vitamin A 10% • Vitamin C 10% • Calcium 20% • Iron 6%
Vitamin D 25% • Vitamin E 15% • Vitamin B6 15%
Folic Acid 10% • Vitamin B12 10%

MILK, WATER, SUGAR, COCOA POWDER, LESS THAN 2% - COCOA POWDER PROCESSED WITH ALKALI, SOY STEROL ESTERS, VITAMINS AND MINERALS [CALCIUM (CALCIUM CHELATE), VITAMIN C (SODIUM ASCORBATE), VITAMIN E (VITAMIN E ACETATE), VITAMIN A (VITAMIN A PALMITATE), VITAMIN D3, VITAMIN B6 (PYRIDOXINE HCL), FOLIC ACID, VITAMIN B12 (CYANOCOBALAMIN)], SOY LECITHIN, POTASSIUM PHOSPHATES, SODIUM POLYPHOSPHATE, CARRAGEENAN, CELLULOSE GEL, CELLULOSE GUM, NATURAL FLAVORS, SALT.

FIGURE 5.3   COCOAVIA NUTRITION FACTS LABEL.

purpose of healthy chocolate. On the opposite end of the spectrum is the CocoaVia Chocolate Snack Bar, with half the amount of sugar as the milk chocolate bar.

The CocoaVia line also has a drink, the CocoaVia Rich Chocolate Indulgence Beverage. Each bottle is 5.65 ounces and contains 24 grams (6 teaspoons) of sugar (see Figure 5.3).

A half-can of Coca-Cola (6 ounces) has 20 grams (5 teaspoons) of sugar. As mentioned, the Kuma Indians drink 3 to 4 cups per day of their cocoa drink to enjoy the antioxidant benefits. To get the same amount of antioxidants from CocoaVia, a person would have to drink approximately 5 ½ CocoaVia Rich Chocolate Indulgence Beverages per day. That would amount to 132 grams of sugar (33 teaspoons) every day, or about three full 12-ounce cans of Coca-Cola.

Even Without Sugar, Chocolate Has Its Negatives

There are reasons (besides sugar) not to eat chocolate, no matter what the chocolate companies say. A major one is caffeine. Caffeine is one of many substances that cause the pancreas to release insulin, a hormone that affects glucose metabolism. If you keep your insulin levels in homeostasis, you're less likely to have insulin problems. Your body will be happier and healthier. However, consuming too much caffeine causes the pancreas to release too much insulin. When this happens, your pancreas is being overworked, and an overworked pancreas is a sure way to increase your risk of getting sick with diabetes.

Caffeine is also a diuretic, which means it makes people go to the bathroom more easily and frequently. This can lead to dehydration, because extra amounts of water leech out of the body between excess urination and defecation. Other effects of caffeine include sleep loss, miscarriages, headaches, jittery nerves, and fatigue. The Center for Science in the Public Interest lists caffeine on its website as something to cut back to minimal levels.[47] Semi-sweet chocolate, which is dark chocolate with a lower sugar amount, has .02 grams of caffeine per ounce. It sounds like chocolate isn't so bad until you realize that very few people eat chocolate only one ounce at a time. Each person is different and the same amount of caffeine can affect people in different ways. As I mentioned in Chapter 3 (page 21), a very small change in chemical or mineral composition can have big results. Therefore, the small amount of caffeine in chocolate (combined with the fact that almost no one eats chocolate one ounce at a time) can certainly affect us in a negative way.

Chocolate also has significant levels of anandamide, which is a naturally occurring chemical that mimics tetrahydrocannabol (THC), better known as marijuana. Now, actually getting high off of chocolate is a losing proposition, since a 130-pound person would need to eat 25 pounds of chocolate to feel the effects of a single joint. However, pot smokers are aware of something called the "pot munchies," which is when the smoker proceeds to eat all kinds of sugary, greasy, and salty foods without regard to the consequences. The anandamide in chocolate can cause a similar "chocolate munchie" effect, which has been linked to bulimia.[48] Bulimia is characterized by food binges that show a preference for high-fat and high-sugar foods, typically chocolate and ice cream. Unfortunately, the bulimic does more than just have the munchies or binge. A person with bulimia also purges, which means they make themselves throw up.

Chocolate also contains phenylethylamine. The body makes and releases this chemical when we are in love. This may explain part of the addictiveness of chocolate and why chocolate is highly associated with romance. One of the reasons so many women love chocolate is because it really is a mood elevator. However, phenylethylamine can cause pulse rate increases and migraines in a person attempting to withdraw from chocolate.

Problems about chocolate seem to keep coming up. For example, chocolate is a highly allergenic food. The reason that chocolate is so allergenic is because we eat it with so much sugar that we have made ourselves allergic to it. As you now know, sugar upsets the body's chemistry and any food that is in the digestive tract at the time of sugar consumption will not digest well, resulting in partially digested foods. The partially digested foods then slip into the bloodstream and can cause an allergic reaction.

Irritability and Lower Bone Density

The *American Journal of Perinatology* presents a case of a mother who ate a lot of chocolate during her pregnancy and while she was nursing her baby. The baby cried excessively and became irritable, jittery, and loud. The mother stopped eating the chocolate and the baby's behavior improved.[49] The researchers believed it was the caffeine in chocolate that caused the child's behavior, but I am not so sure. It might have been the chocolate itself, since all people react differently to different foods.

In January 2008, a study from the University of Western Australia School of Medicine and Pharmacology focused on whether the flavanols in chocolate would help improve calcium absorption into bones. The researcher expected it would. The study focused on women between the ages of seventy and eighty-five. The results were not what the researcher expected. They showed that the more chocolate or cocoa consumed, the lower the women's bone densities were, as measured by x-ray.[50]

Researchers haven't been able to figure out why. It's like they don't have a clue that the sugar in chocolate is leeching the calcium out of bones, upsetting body chemistry, and making chocolate eaters allergic to chocolate. Flavanols and other similar antioxidants can be found in other foods, though they are more prevalent in chocolate. If you're looking for an alternative source of antioxidants, you can try consuming moderate amounts of onions, red wine, tea, apples, or raspberries. Flavanols also come in capsule form, which don't have the sugar, fat, or anything else in chocolate that may harm you.

Look, if you just have to have the chocolate goodness, you're going to increase your chances of dying early. Unless, of course, you want to find raw chocolate, mix it with Jalapeño peppers, and see if Montezuma actually knew what he was talking about. That original recipe is something we can refer to as a taste of character—a person has nothing left to prove when it comes to being brave enough to drink the Aztec chocolate. Come on, drink it. It's just chocolate. No, you do it first. I made the dare first.

However, if you're like me, you'll wisely decline this dare and simply not eat any chocolate, because the processing and added sugar makes store-bought chocolate difficult for the body to digest.

CONCLUSION

Hopefully this chapter has helped you realize that this glut of sugar that we eat upsets the body chemistry, leading to a host of diseases that you will read about in the next chapter. Whole, unprocessed foods with no added sugar are the best foods for you. Let us always eat food that is "yummy, yummy, in our tummies."

6

Sugar-Related Diseases and Conditions

There are many diseases and conditions that are related to sugar intake, with sugar not only causing but continuing the progression of some diseases. In this chapter, I have emphasized diseases that are most prevalent in our society. Most people do not relate these diseases to sugar. For example, the medical community relates obesity to overeating. Yes, that is true, but what causes overeating? You got it—sugar.

You will learn that eating too much sugar can sometimes lead to hypoglycemia (low blood sugar), and that contrary to what you may believe, eating more sugar won't help stabilize your blood sugar. Information on the diseases and problems sugar can cause in children will help you stop the sugar addiction early in your own children's lives.

Sometimes, the medical community calls a disease a "syndrome," which consists of many symptoms and diseases. I have written about the metabolic syndrome. Some of the symptoms and diseases related to this syndrome include elevated triglycerides, raised cholesterol, high fasting blood glucose levels, high blood pressure, elevated low-density lipoproteins, and elevated insulin levels. In this instance, I am speaking about more than one disease. Other diseases that show a great relationship to sugar will surprise you, such as dementia and cancer.

I have seen the negative effects of sugar all over the world, and I am giving you a brief look at my findings. The western diet is making its mark on far too many places.

Finally, sugar can also lead to convulsive, reoccurring seizures, a disease known as epilepsy.

Of course, unmentioned ailments and diseases are not immune to sugar's unhealthy effects. Including every disease affected by sugar would take up far too much space, which is why I've decided to focus on some of the main ones here. For a much more detailed list of why sugar is ruining your health, see Chapter 2 (page 13). Be wary of what you eat—as you'll learn, the diseases that result from overindulging are not worth the temporary satisfaction you get from that sugary meal or snack.

OBESITY: THE FATTENING OF AMERICA

I'm sure you've heard that obesity is on the rise in America. So just how fat are Americans, anyway? In 2002, researchers reported average BMI statistics for men and women. To refresh, a person's BMI is a measurement of his or her body fat based on height and weight. (To find out how to calculate your BMI, go to page 44.) According to BMI guidelines, a BMI ranging between 25 and 29.9 indicates that a person is overweight. A BMI of 30 or above is considered obese. The study showed that women weighed in with an average BMI of 27.8, but men dominated at 28.2.[1]

Clearly, Americans are doing a toe dance with obesity. The National Heart, Lung, and Blood Institute (NHLBI) used government statistics for height and weight to determine that men and women gained an average of ten pounds each between 1998 and 2002.

Another way to look at the problem is to measure the circumference of the waist. Healthy sizes have been determined to be less than 34 inches for a woman and less than 38 inches for a man. A study conducted in 2002 showed that the average woman had a waist circumference of 36.5 inches, while men bloated out at 39 inches.

At those sizes, both women and men move into the realm of a serious problem. We have some leeway with BMI, but according to circumference, the average woman and man are already obese.[2]

What Causes Obesity?

We continue to gain weight because of the related effects of our sedentary lifestyles. We have machines to do the work we used to have to do ourselves, whether it was walking the golf course or washing clothes. The level of naturally-occurring exercise has dropped. Now, neither my staff nor I are machine-hating Luddites by any stretch of the imagination. This book was written using several Apple MacBooks. That being said, our workday does involve—for most of us—sitting and processing information via computer screens.

Then, many of us go home to sit in front of the TV to receive our entertainment. This creates an interesting cycle where people have a tendency to overeat foods that are easy and convenient to prepare—we don't want to miss the key clue that will help solve the mystery by the last commercial break or the twist at the end of our favorite TV show. Most foods eaten while watching TV are artificially sweetened and easy to take out of a wrapper, because cutting up a salad takes time.

It's not just an inactive lifestyle that leads to obesity. There are three hormones—leptin, ghrelin, and insulin—that deal with fullness, hunger, and sugar metabolism. They may help explain why we get fat when we thoughtlessly eat in front of the TV (or at our desks, or anywhere). Leptin tells the body it is full. Ghrelin tells the body it is hungry. Insulin metabolizes most sugars. Leptin and ghrelin play directly opposite each other.

Insulin removes excess blood glucose from the bloodstream by taking it to the cells that need energy. However, a high blood sugar environment combined with little-to-no exercise means that a lot of glucose will be converted into fat. An insulin release is the primary mechanism of telling the body to make less ghrelin to make you feel full. On the surface, it seems like a simple answer would be to exercise more. However, there are people who work out very hard and still get nowhere—except, maybe, more hungry.

Diet and Exercise Won't Always Do the Trick

Not all sweeteners and sugars respond to the insulin cycle. For example, fructose doesn't use insulin to metabolize. It metabolizes in the liver. Therefore, no insulin is released when we eat fructose, so ghrelin levels remain constant and the body still feels hungry.[3] According to the U.S. Census Bureau, consumption of high fructose corn syrup increased from 19 pounds per person per year in 1980 to 63.8 pounds per person per year in 2000.[4] Since fructose causes people to keep feeling hungry even after eating, they are likely to continue eating until obesity eventually sets in. [5,6] (For more on fructose, see Fructose Roulette on page 60.)

Unfortunately, many mainstream health practitioners assume that motivating their patients to diet and exercise is all that needs to happen to make the patients thinner, if not actually thin. They are laboring under years of misinformation, possibly created by Big Sugar, that say sugar is only a problem for dentists. I have always wondered why people don't question that if sugar makes holes in very hard tissues in your body (your teeth), what does it do to the soft tissues?

Part of the reason for this is that obese people have been known to underreport their food and sugar intake. For many years, based on people's self-reporting of sugar consumption, researchers have said that sugar is not a factor in obesity. Then researchers found that urinary sugar excretion, in twenty-four hour urine collections, can serve as an independent marker of sugar consumption. To test this, the researchers has test subjects submit all of their urine collected over a twenty-four hour period. They found that when obese people had a high urinary secretion of sugar, it did not correlate with the sugar intake that they reported eating. In normal-weight people, the findings were similar. Researchers understand now that sugar plays a huge role in obesity.[7] This concept reinforces the old adage from Alcoholics Anonymous: How can you tell when an addict is lying? He opens his mouth.

Health practitioners will agree that sugar and other sweeteners have only one purpose: adding calories to your diet. They don't always make the leap of thought that if a food only adds calories and no other nutrients, then maybe that food can safely be replaced in our diets by complex carbohydrates or protein and vegetables.

Studies on Sugar Addiction and Obesity

As you learned in Chapter 1, sugar is addictive. To take that thought one step further--sugar is an addictive substance that can lead to obesity. It is possible to be thin and addicted to sugar, but not probable. Some sugar addicts binge and purge to stay thin. If they binge but don't purge, they either skip meals or spend half of their days exercising to avoid gaining weight.[8]

There is research showing that obesity and also addiction can start in the womb. While studying this concept, researchers fed a healthy diet of rat chow to some rats and an unhealthy diet of rat food and junk food to other rats while the rats were pregnant or lactating. The junk food consisted of sugary, fatty, and salty foods. The primary thrust of the study was to figure out if what the mama rat ate during pregnancy and lactation affected the food preferences and obesity risks of her offspring.

The rats exposed to the unhealthy diets preferred consuming sugar water above anything else, even when healthier options were available. The results showed that for the most part, after birth, the baby rats largely made the same food choices their mothers did.

The babies born to the sugar-eating mothers were not heavier at birth than the ones born to the healthy-eating mothers, but they gained weight at near astronomical rates as they approached adulthood. Their choice of food was similar to their mother's diet while she was pregnant and lactating. It follows that while rats and humans are different, many studies can translate between species.[9]

Dr. Jeffrey Gordon of Washington University in St. Louis and his group of researchers have been conducting ongoing studies on weight gain since the 1990s. The results fascinate me. The team used mice as their subjects. They found that a certain type of intestinal bacteria in the mice may have been causing weight gain. The dominant bacteria in the gut of obese mice were Firmicutes. Mice that were thin had more Bacteroidetes in their system. Firmicutes have more genes for breaking down complex starches and fiber. When you break down the complex carbohydrates easily, you add calories and can gain weight. Bacteroidetes are not as efficient at breaking down fiber and complex carbohydrates and therefore, mice with Bacteroidetes in their systems do not digest as much, meaning they don't absorb as many calories. Therefore, they stay thinner. When Firmicutes were transplanted into the lean mice, the mice gained weight.[10]

Parallel to the mouse study results, the researchers also found that heavy humans had far more Firmicutes bacteria than thinner humans. They then asked their overweight subjects to go on a low-fat, low-refined carbohydrate diet for one year. As the test subjects lost weight, the bacteria in their stomachs changed from Firmicutes to predominantly Bacteroidetes. It appears that obesity itself contributes to an increase in fat storage via a change in the ratio of bacteria. In this research, it certainly shows that calories don't count by themselves. Remove the sugar, fat, and excess weight, and you will not absorb all the calories you consume.[11]

It would be a good idea if you are overweight and want to get pregnant to get back to your normal weight first. This will give your baby a chance to grow up without a weight problem. But it is still important to control what you put in your mouth and your baby's mouth—at any weight.

The future of obesity looks grim. According to a study at the Johns Hopkins Bloomberg School of Public Health's Center for Human Nutrition, 75 percent of adults and 24 percent of children and adolescents in the United States will be overweight or obese by the year 2015.

The study combined the results of twenty prior studies and four national surveys. They found that the portion of the population that is overweight or obese has increased by an average of .3 to .8 percent per year since the 1960s. In the 1960s, 13 percent of the population was obese. The percentage increased to 32 percent by 2004. The researchers project that by 2015, the percentage of obese people will reach 41 percent. Among children and adolescents, 16 percent are currently overweight, while 34 percent are at risk.[12] The research also showed that higher rates of obesity are found among groups with lower educational and income levels, among racial and ethnic minorities, and in high-poverty areas.

Putting an End to Obesity

Dieters should focus on limiting the amount of fructose they eat instead of cutting out starchy foods like bread, rice, and potatoes. Dr. Richard Johnson at the University of Florida at Gainsville proposed using new dietary guidelines—based on fructose—to gauge how healthy foods are. Johnson says that potatoes, pasta, and rice may be relatively safe to eat when compared to table sugar.[13] I agree completely. Potatoes, pasta, and rice do not suppress the immune system, and fructose does.

Portion sizes are a definite key to obesity control. Plate sizes have increased every year since 1982. The *Journal of the American Dietetic Association* found interesting information. A study demonstrated that current portion sizes are larger than standard portions developed by the U.S. Department of Agriculture (USDA) in 1982. The mean weight of muffins (6 $1/2$ ounces) was more than three times the weight of the USDA's standards. The mean weight of cookies (4 ounces) was eight times that of USDA's "medium" cookie. For most foods, the smallest size available was larger than USDA's standards.[14]

If you gradually reduce the amount of food you put on your plate, you will start seeing some results on the scale. The idea is to lose weight gradually. Food Plan III (see page 112) is good for weight reduction. Use this plan with four or five small portions a day and you will see results.

Drastically reducing your intake of sweeteners will also help. I always come back to sugar as the primary cause of ill health. I have already shown the correlation between obese people and sugar. However, it's important to remember that sugar is an addiction, and therefore must be broken slowly.

Depending on the severity of obesity and other health problems, your health practitioner may recommend taking brisk walks of up to one hour between three and five times a week. You will also have to change your diet. On the contrary, if the only thing you do is remove all forms of sugar from your diet, I am sure you will be pleasantly surprised with the results.

Between 280,000 and 325,000 people die every year from obesity-related ailments.[15] Failure to take action will greatly increase your chances of becoming obese and joining this statistic. I trust you'll choose wisely.

I thought we should end this section with a prayer by actor Victor Buono.

"Fat Man's Prayer"

by Victor Buono

Lord, My soul is ripped with riot
incited by my wicked diet.
"We Are What We Eat," said a wise old man!
And, Lord, if that's true, then I'm a garbage can.

I want to rise on Judgment Day, that's plain!
But at my present weight, I'll need a crane.
So grant me strength, that I may not fall
into the clutches of cholesterol.

May my flesh with carrot-curls be sated,
that my soul may be polyunsaturated.
And show me the light, that I may bear witness
to the President's Council on Physical Fitness.

And at oleomargarine I'll never mutter,
for the road to Hell is spread with butter.
And cream is cursed; and cake is awful;
and Satan is hiding in every waffle.

Mephistopheles lurks in provolone;
the Devil is in each ice cream cone.
Beelzebub is a chocolate drop,
and Lucifer is a lollipop.

Give me this day my daily slice
but, cut it thin and toast it twice.
I beg upon my dimpled knees,
deliver me from Jujubes.

And when my days of trial are done,
and my war with malted milk is won,
Let me stand with the Saints in Heaven
In a shining robe—size 37.

I can do it Lord, If You'll show to me,
the virtues of lettuce and celery.
If You'll teach me the evil of mayonnaise,
of pasta a la Milannaise
potatoes a la Lyonnaise
and crisp-fried chicken from the South.
Lord, if you love me, shut my mouth.

Victor Buono once said, "I think that I shall never see—my feet."
He died in 1982 at age forty-three of a heart attack, weighing more
than 350 pounds.

As you will see in the following sections, consuming too much
sugar can not only lead to obesity, but many other diseases as well.

HYPOGLYCEMIA:
LOW BLOOD SUGAR DOES NOT MEAN EAT MORE SUGAR

I have followed Roberta Ruggario's foundation, the Hypoglycemia Support Foundation, Inc., and her work for over twenty years. After reading her book, *The Do's and Don'ts of Hypoglycemia: An Everyday Guide to Low Blood Sugar,* I felt it was important for Roberta to write a section on hypoglycemia, as she is the expert on this subject. Roberta has a passion for teaching people about hypoglycemia, just like I have a passion for teaching people about sugar. So, here is an article written by an expert who, like me, just wants to share her information.

Hypoglycemia and Sugar:
Is There a Correlation?

You see, I've been there—I've lived through the devastating effects of hypoglycemia and the ignorance of not knowing what sugar can do to the body, both physically and mentally.

It took a life-altering experience to learn why sugar is labeled by some as the white plague, the quiet killer, and the most destructive, addictive chemical of choice. It has been written that it causes fatal diseases, contributes to our nation's crime and delinquency, and may be at the root of most mental and emotional problems. Perhaps the late Dr. Harvey Ross said it the best when he wrote in his book, Hypoglycemia: The Disease Your Doctor Won't Treat, that, "The difference between eating natural, unrefined carbohydrates and refined sugar can be the difference between life and death, for refined sugar is lethal when ingested by human beings."

As a young mother, I had no idea of sugar's consequences. I lived on Yankee Doodles, Devil Dogs, hot fudge sundaes, and hot apple pies. I would swing from not eating meals to eating high-carbohydrate ones that consisted of pasta and bread. It was no wonder I had chronic fatigue and couldn't get up in the morning, insomnia where it was hard to go to sleep at night, headaches that felt like my head was going to explode, and depression that made me ask myself, "Am I going crazy?"

That scenario lasted ten years (from 1960–1970), during which time I faced dozens of doctors, countless tests, thousands of pills, and even the administration of electric shock therapy—only to be told I had a severe case of functional hypoglycemia (also known as low blood sugar) and that all I needed was a diet! Yes, a simple glucose tolerance test, proper diagnosis, and an elimination of sugar finally lead me down the road to recovery. What is so sad is that what happened to me almost forty years ago is still happening to people today. It should be noted that forty years ago the only test for blood glucose problems was the glucose tolerance test. Today there are other less invasive tests that a person can take to test for hypoglycemia or hyperglycemia. Read about these in the section on blood sugar problems on page 38.

I receive almost 500 e-mails a month from all over the world through my website, www.hypoglycemia.org. This is an extension of the Hypoglycemia Support Foundation, Inc. (HSF). I founded HSF in 1980 to give information, support, hope, and encouragement to those suffering from hypoglycemia, something that was lacking when I was sick and had nowhere to turn.

My message is simple. Your symptoms may not be in your head. If you suffer from fatigue, insomnia, mental confusion, nervousness, mood swings, faintness, headaches, depression, phobias, blurred vision, inner trembling, outbursts of temper, sudden hunger, heart palpitations, cravings for sweets, allergies, and crying spells (just to name a few), you may have functional hypoglycemia—most likely a result of poor diet, stress, and lifestyle.

I would like to elaborate here for just a moment. For me, personally, it was a change of diet that was life-altering. But it soon became evident that stress and lifestyle also play a major role in controlling hypoglycemia symptoms. You can't be on the perfect diet and go to work every day to a job you hate. You won't be completely happy. You can't eat perfectly balanced meals and exercise five to six hours a day. It isn't fathomable. And you won't succeed at anything if you tell yourself "this won't" or "this can't" work. Above all, if you're addicted to nicotine, caffeine, or alcohol, you need to know that all these substances will trigger or worsen existing hypoglycemia. So, whether you are dealing with a blood sugar imbalance or any kind of illness, healing the whole body is an absolute must—physically, mentally, emotionally, and spiritually. This shouldn't frighten you. Just take one day, one step at a time—and interweave it with education, commitment, application, and love.

So, what exactly is hypoglycemia? And what role does sugar play? To really understand the process easily and effortlessly, I asked Dr. Lorna Walker, HSF's nutritionist for the past twenty-five years, for her input. This is what she had to say:

"Seale Harris, MD, first described reactive or functional hypoglycemia in 1924. He, appropriately, labeled it hyperinsulinism. Today, the terms reactive hypoglycemia, functional hypoglycemia, and idiopathic hyperinsulinism are used interchangeably.

"In hypoglycemia, the pancreas is supersensitive to rapid rises in blood glucose and responds by secreting too much insulin. But does this mean that eating sugar causes hypoglycemia? There have been few studies on the relationship between sugar and refined carbohydrate consumption and the development of hypoglycemia. There is, however, empirical evidence to strongly suggest there is a correlation.

"The most obvious is the dietary therapy for hypoglycemia. Patients with hypoglycemia are helped by a diet low in sugars and refined carbohydrates (which are rapidly turned into sugar). By avoiding what sets the pancreas off, the hypoglycemia is controlled. Since the average American consumes nearly 150 pounds of sugar each year, it is reasonable to assume that many will succumb to this constant attack on the pancreas by developing reactive hypoglycemia.

"Next, there is the increasing number of type-2 diabetics . . . being diagnosed each year. Children as young as twelve years old are now being diagnosed with this condition. Type-2 diabetics have elevated insulin levels, just like people with functional hypoglycemia. However, their cells no longer respond to insulin's message. Obesity plays a role in this scenario, yet we know insulin facilitates fat storage and more insulin facilitates more fat storage. Is it not reasonable to conclude that the constant consumption of sugar-laden, highly-refined foods ultimately exhausts the pancreas until it can no longer control blood glucose levels? I believe it is. Dr. Harris was quoted as saying, 'The low blood sugar of today is the diabetes of tomorrow.'

"The treatment for type-2 diabetes is weight loss (to decrease the insulin insensitivity) and essentially the exact same diet used to treat hypoglycemia. With such common sense evidence pointing to a dietary cause for hypoglycemia, it is time to implore the scientific community to perform the epidemiological studies needed to prove it!"

So, whether you have been diagnosed as having hypoglycemia or just think you have it, the first requirement is education. Learn as much as you can about this condition, and then, as a knowledgeable patient, you will be able to wisely choose a healthcare professional who can assist you with your diagnosis and treatment. Congratulate yourself—you're now on the road to recovery.

Many thanks to Roberta. Her article is full of important information. Food Plan III (see page 112) is the perfect diet for a person with
low blood sugar problems. You can use this food plan and eat small
portions four or five times a day to get yourself back on track. This
is important for people with hypoglycemia and will help keep their
blood sugar stabilized. Use the Body Monitor Kit (see page 182 for
ordering information) to find out the foods to which your body is
sensitive. Foods to which you are allergic can raise or lower your
blood sugar levels out of the normal range, resulting in consequences
you should avoid.

Sugar Is Not a Toy

"Sugar and spice and everything nice, that's what little girls are made of."
This nursery rhyme about the unscientific composition of little girls may
hold mountains of information for a future sociologist about gender
expectations during the bad old days, whenever they were (or are). Girls
and women have traditionally been homemakers, so naturally, a magical
process causes pastry ingredients to become part of their bodies. However, in actual practice, the rhyme is wrong—boys are made of sugar, too.

Statistically, teenage boys lead all other gender and age groups for
average consumption of sugar and other sweeteners, clocking in at one
cup per day.[16] But children of all types aren't very far behind, so a lot of
people have a problem—or will soon.

Sugar enters the picture early. Many newborn babies receive an IV
bottle that is 5 percent glucose before going home from the hospital.
Some baby formulas, such as Enfamil, Pro Sobec Lipil, and Similac Go &
Grow still have a form of sugar or high fructose corn syrup. Read your
labels carefully and phone the manufacturer for more information. Don't
be fooled by Similac Organic, which has evaporated sugarcane. There are
formulas out there without any form of sugar. Calm Nat Baby Formula is
one. Tell your healthcare provider your concern and ask his or her advice.

Sugar is an addiction that starts early as we grow up eating what our
parents eat. Unhealthy parents can have unhealthy children, because parents have the ability to pass their unhealthy eating habits on to their kids,
thus starting the child's sugar addiction in the womb. A rat study conducted in London showed that pregnant and lactating rats that ate high-
sugar diets produced offspring that preferred junk food themselves. The

mother rats gained enormous amounts of weight as they ate high-sugar foods, but the offspring who had lapped the diet up in their mothers' milk were even more obese.

With habits like these, how can we not expect our kids to grow up hooked on sweets?

This chapter is about diseases caused by sugar, and even though this section is not about a specific disease per se, it is still important to understand the various effects giving sugar to our kids can have.

Needless to say, we have to stop feeding our children sugar.

Sugar Affects Kids Worse Than Adults

Sugar may be worse for kids than it is for adults because kids react so strongly and with much wilder swings of body chemistry. Some of their body systems are not fully developed. The immune system is still developing the acquired immunity to fight off infections, and the digestive system must learn to handle the variety of foods in our diet.

A child's body is learning and working continually, and sugar just causes it to work harder. At least children have the ability to snap back to homeostasis much quicker than adults, because children haven't yet trained their bodies to enjoy sugar's abuse. These body chemistry changes not only cause physical ailments, such as allergies and asthma, but have also, in many studies, put children on a roller coaster of emotional effects that include hyperactivity, aggressiveness, sadness, low self-esteem, mania, sleepiness, and many more.

There are several approaches to explain how sugar affects the emotions and the mind. One put forth by Dr. William Crook in his article, "Why Does the Ingestion of Sugar Cause Hyperactivity in Many Children?" points to Candida Albicans, a yeast that needs sugar in order to thrive. An immune system depression, which I have discussed many times in this book, allows Candida to multiply unchecked in the body. In one study, a rat that was fed dextrose had a 200 percent higher incidence of Candida growths in its gastrointestinal tract than ones who were not fed dextrose. Many researchers studying Candida have noted a higher degree of gut permeability in people who have it. This may allow undigested food into the bloodstream. The body's reaction to these invasive particles releases chemicals that can affect emotions.[17]

I think there are more ways sugar can change emotional states. My research has mostly centered on mineral relationships that, when knocked out of balance, can wreak havoc with enzyme and hormone production in the body. This process can include the neurotransmitters, which tell the body what to think and feel, and testosterone, which is linked to aggressiveness.

Other Side Effects Sugar Has On Kids

Obesity is certainly a good reason to wean kids from sugar, since it is increasing rapidly in children. But, the main reason to nix the sugar we feed our kids is type-2 diabetes, which is increasing in children, not type-1 diabetes, which is the usual type of diabetes children get.

The Differences Between Type-1 and Type-2 Diabetes

Type-1 diabetes, once known as "juvenile" or "insulin-dependent" diabetes, is a chronic condition in which the pancreas produces little or no insulin. Although type-1 diabetes can develop at any age, it typically appears during childhood or adolescence. The medical community believes that this type of diabetes is either genetic or caused by a virus. Despite active research, type-1 diabetes has no cure. Less than 10 percent of all diabetics are type-1.

Type-2 diabetes is much more common. It is a condition in which the body becomes resistant to the effects of insulin, even though it may be producing enough insulin. Or, the body produces some, but not enough, insulin to maintain a normal blood sugar level. Treatment for type-2 diabetes revolves around varied combinations of diet, exercise, medications, and insulin injections. Many people do not require insulin injections once they have changed some lifestyle factors. Over 90 percent of diabetics are type-2.

Both types of diabetes can be helped with diet, many times dramatically. To help deal with food allergies and foods your body is not processing well, immediately go on Food Plan III (see page 112) and use the Body Monitoring Kit (ordering information is on page 182) to test.

The Scientific (and Anecdotal) Proof

When we consider the mental and emotional effects sugar has on children, perhaps one small reason as to why some of our educational systems fail becomes clear. Children who are affected by sugar can have a hard time concentrating, or they can become sleepy or hyperactive.

These symptoms can affect school grades and school advancement. For the first time in U.S. history, your child is less likely to graduate from high school than you were. Out of every four kids, one is dropping out of high school. Among minority students, more than one out of every three students will drop out of high school before graduation.[18]

Reducing the amount of sugar kids receive in school has done wonders in the past and is doing wonders today. The following story will make you smile, and for those of you with elementary school children, I hope you contact Healthy Kids, Smart Kids (see Resources, page 144).

In 1998, Yvonne Sanders-Butler became principal of Browns Mill Elementary School in Lithonia, Georgia. At that time, 20 percent of her students were overweight and many students ate a "typical" breakfast—a doughnut, candy, or a soft drink—or they ate nothing. Some 300 students had filed excuses not to participate in gym. The state academic tests were only passed by just over 50 percent of the students.

With the approval of the PTA, Sanders-Butler banned all candy, soft drinks, and sugary snacks from cafeteria and brown-bag lunches. Each day, all lunches and snacks are inspected, and sugary treats are replaced with a banana or apple. All the students and their parents sign a wellness pledge, and those who stick to the program win homework passes and other prizes. Today, at Brown Mills Elementary School, there is not a single obese child and 80 percent of the students pass the state tests. As of September 2008, seventeen other schools around the United States have joined the program, which is called Healthy Kids, Smart Kids. Sanders-Butler is now working with the Robert Wood Johnson Foundation to help spread the word.[19]

The problem extends to other countries, too. In Norway, where soft drink consumption averages 30 gallons per person per year, a questionnaire went out to more than 5,000 tenth graders. In the study, 45 percent of boys and 21 percent of girls admitted to drinking more than one glass of soda per day. The questions sought to relate levels of soda consumption to school conduct problems and many common mental health indicators, like anxiety, hyperactivity, dizzy spells, hopelessness, panic, sadness, low self-esteem, insomnia, and a sense of feeling weighed down by burdens. Kids who drank four or more soft drinks per day scored the highest for hyperactivity and overall behavioral and mental problems. The rates decreased with lower soft drink consumption.[20] (For more about eating habits in other countries, see Faraway Places, page 101.)

The study put forth some additional ideas that couldn't be tested with just a questionnaire. The researchers noted that the high calorie content in soda could cause a student to feel full and in turn skip meals with nutrient-rich foods. Nutrient-rich foods help stabilize blood sugar, and they contain nutrients such as iron and protein, which can affect emotional states.

Other researchers and I have linked sugar to most maladies in adults not inflicted by gunshots or hard falls. (Turn back to page 13 and read 140 Reasons Why Sugar is Ruining Your Health to find out the significance of that statement.) Many people might make the logical assumption that what is bad for adults can't be good for kids, and they would be correct in doing so.

What studies do exist are, unfortunately, contradictory. As of yet, no truly definitive science exists to make the link between kids' emotional states and their sugary diets. The few studies I've mentioned supporting that hypothesis are a good start, but some studies have surfaced that show no relationship between the two, counteracting the numerous ones that do. However, I'll ask you to put science aside for a minute and consider the anecdotal evidence we can see with our own eyes. Over the years, kids have gotten heavier. They've gotten lazier. They've been more inclined to act out with bad behavior. I'm sure you've noticed some of these observations.

How many times has the cranky child in Target, demanding every toy in sight, been described as being coked up on sugar? And when you were with a child who was acting out, how many of those times had the child consumed a Coke, candy bar, or Ding Dong within the previous two hours? How many times have you acted out because you felt lousy and wanted sugar?

We can see with our own eyes what sugar can do to children. We know what the problem is—the difficult part is the solution.

Removing Sugar From Our Kids' Diets

Sugar addiction is far tougher to overcome than any other addiction, and our society doesn't help. Most of our holidays have been invented by greeting card and candy companies. Sugary holidays abound: Valentine's Day, Easter, Halloween, Christmas, Thanksgiving, Fourth of July, and Hanukkah are all holidays that would not be complete without sweets and baking.

Let's not forget the ritual of the Girl Scout Cookies, church bake sales, and the average child's birthday party. And then, kids grow up with soda.

Sugar is bad for people, especially kids. So what now? How do we remove sugar from our kids' diets?

In my experience, it starts with parents evaluating their own sugar intake and cutting back themselves. I couldn't get my own kids, ages seven and eleven when I started, to even think about eliminating sugar until I cut back myself. Among other benefits, my mood improved by doing this. I believe that the psychologically healthier home life I created may have helped my kids. I think I set a right example that helped them make good decisions about sugar and all food.

I didn't make my kids go cold turkey. I would let them have one dessert per day for a little while before phasing out desserts entirely. On Halloween, I would let them eat a small handful of candy and throw the rest out. It was only after my kids stopped trick-or-treating that I thought to give them presents as a tradeoff for their candy.

Needless to say, I banned soft drinks in the house from the jump.

My kids did eat sugar outside the house and I said very little because I didn't want to harp about the sugar I didn't see. Too much enforcement can cause an opposite, rebellious reaction in kids. But, for my part, I wouldn't buy them any sugary foods, nor would I keep any in my house.

My studies also led me to some interesting educational tools that may go a long way in persuading kids to give up sugar. You could have your kids read you the labels of the foods they eat and have them tell you how much sugar in grams is in the food. Then, you could use the conversion of 4 grams equals 1 teaspoon and have your kids pour the sugar into a glass cup just to see how much of it they eat. I also believe that instead of rewarding good behavior with a sugary treat, small trinkets (such as balloons, crayons, or other knickknacks from the 99-cent store) do the job just fine. My daughter came up with a great idea for Halloween. Instead of giving candy and other sugary junk food, she gives trick-or-treaters glow in the dark bracelets sold on the Internet.

If your child has any of the following problems, I suggest that you take sugar completely out of his or her diet for at least ten days.

- Allergies

- Cannot go for more than four hours without eating

- Colds or bacterial infections more than once a year

- Difficulty concentrating
- Difficulty falling asleep or staying asleep
- Frequent headaches
- Hyperactivity or listlessness
- Low grades in school
- Many dental fillings
- Overweight

You have nothing to lose. In fact, you will probably save a lot of money not buying soft drinks, ice cream, cakes, candy, and the like. You might even alleviate some symptoms your child is having and help his or her health. Early childhood symptoms can mean adult degenerative diseases.

However, keep in mind that not all problems with kids are dietary, so removing sugar from the diet isn't necessarily a fix-all solution. It's worth a shot, but being supportive about other things going on in your child's life is still necessary.

You can control what your child eats in your home, so start now.

METABOLIC SYNDROME: TOUGH SUBJECT, EASY ANSWER

It seems like doctors just love to name things with multi-syllable words, and "syndrome" is a favorite, designed to scare people. In the case of metabolic syndrome, perhaps we should be concerned. It is estimated that between 25 and 50 percent of American adults have it or may get it.[21]

Metabolic syndrome is characterized by a group of metabolic risk factors.[22] One study suggests that if you have three of the following criteria, you may have metabolic syndrome:

- Elevated blood pressure (at least 130 systolic over 90 diastolic).
- Elevated C-reactive protein, which signifies inflammation in the bloodstream.
- High fasting blood glucose levels (110 mg/dL or higher).
- High triglycerides (over 150 mg/dL).
- A large waistline (39 inches for men and 36.5 inches for women).[23]

- Low levels of high-density lipoprotein (HDL), (under 40 mg/dL in men and under 50 mg/dL in women).

- Raised low-density lipoprotein (LDL) levels (over 150 mg/dL).

- Raised total cholesterol levels (over 200 mg/dL).

If you have three or more of these symptoms, it would be wise to be checked by a health practitioner.

Insulin Resistance

Some of the metabolic syndrome symptoms have been discussed already, but let's take a minute to define the biggie—insulin resistance. Years of highly refined dietary carbohydrate intake (especially in genetically-predisposed individuals) stress insulin receptors, which, in turn, malfunction.

There are other factors that contribute to becoming insulin-resistant, as well. Smoking is one of them. Smoking cigarettes increases insulin resistance and worsens the health consequences of metabolic syndrome. If you smoke, add this to the list of reasons why you should quit.[24]

In a person with normal metabolism, insulin is released from the pancreas after eating sugar and signals insulin-sensitive muscle and fat tissues in the body. The muscle and fat tissues absorb the sugar to lower the blood glucose to a normal level. This brings the glucose level back to homeostasis.

In an insulin-resistant person, however, normal levels of insulin do not trigger the signal for glucose absorption by muscle and fat cells. To compensate for this, an insulin-resistant individual's pancreas releases much more insulin than it should so that the cells can absorb the glucose. Higher levels of insulin can often control blood glucose levels adequately, at least for a while. This resistance can take place with both the body's own insulin and through insulin injection.

Other lesser-known effects of insulin have recently come into play. They include:

- Elevated C-reactive protein, which indicates inflammation.

- Elevated serum triglycerides.

- Enhanced synthesis of cholesterol, thus raising the cholesterol level in the bloodstream.

- Encouraging storage rather than burning of fat, thus leading to obesity.

- High insulin levels.

- Increasing secretion of norepinephrine, which can increase blood pressure and pulse rate.

- Increasing the tendency to form blood clots.[25]

- Leading to glycation, which is when glucose binds with protein non-enzymatically and can lead to cataracts, wrinkles, and other problems.

- Lowering your levels of high-density lipoproteins (HDL), which increases the risk of heart disease.

- Raising the low-density lipoproteins (LDL) in the bloodstream, which increases the risk of vascular disease.

- Retaining sodium (salt), resulting in a subsequent rise in blood pressure.

- Stimulating your brain and liver to make you hungry and manufacture fat.

- Thickening arterial walls, which makes blood vessels more stiff, leading to increased blood pressure and increased risk of vascular disease.

- Type-2 diabetes.

- Upsetting hormonal balance. Hormones work in relation to one another, so when one of them increases or decreases, others secrete more of their hormone in order to maintain homeostasis. Insulin goes first, since that is the hormone food comes into contact with first. Thyroid is affected next, followed by pituitary glands, and then the adrenal gland.

High insulin levels can lead to obesity, as noted in the list. Elevated insulin levels have also been called "diabesity," because of the common link between type-2 diabetes and obesity.[26] The problem is worldwide, reaching epidemic proportions in the United States and many developing countries like China and India.[27,28,29] Domestically, incidences of type-2 diabetes rose 765 percent from 1935 to 1966.[30] Worldwide rates are expected to rise 46 percent by 2010, from 150 million to 221 million cases.[31]

Other Connections to Metabolic Syndrome

One study showed that patients with metabolic syndrome increased their risk for oxidative stress, which is linked to heart disease and a lower HDL production, by 3.7 times. As soon as children drink their first high fructose corn syrup soft drink, they increase their risk of developing heart disease as they get older. I've already discussed the specific effects of fructose, but any sugar-rich diet seems to have these effects on metabolic syndrome and heart disease. Children who eat too much sugar and become heavy are more likely to develop heart disease or metabolic syndrome when they get older.[32]

Inflammation also plays a role in developing metabolic syndrome. Inflammatory processes work to make the body safe from injuries, foreign invaders, and allergens. Sugar can cause food allergies through a general depression of the immune system. Inflammation is the byproduct of this process. Inflammation in the bloodstream can be measured by blood tests for C-reactive protein and Interleukin-6.

A five-year study was conducted on older people dealing with cognitive impairment to determine the complex relationship between inflammation and metabolic syndrome. The average age of the participants was seventy-four. The results showed that participants who had metabolic syndrome were more likely to show declines on mental function (memory, confusion, alertness) tests across the board. However, when metabolic syndrome was cross-correlated with high inflammation, the risk for a decline in mental function was at its highest. Elderly people with metabolic syndrome and low inflammation had considerably better results on the mental tests. But, the best performers were the healthy people who did not have metabolic syndrome.[33]

Stress can also play a role in metabolic syndrome, which explains why there is a high correlation between stress reduction and lowering your metabolic syndrome markers. A serious workout punching walls can burn energy and relieve stress (though your bill to hang new drywall may cause new stresses). However, not all people relieve their stress through working out and may need additional forms of stress reduction. A 2006 study into the effects of meditation on the risk factors of metabolic syndrome and heart disease found that sixteen weeks of meditation improved markers significantly.[34] So, this is where I tell you to meditate. Pray. Vent in a journal. Bend yourself into a pretzel position with yoga. Pet your dog. Based on your likes and dislikes, doing even just one of these methods will help reduce stress and lower your risk for metabolic syndrome.

Conquering Metabolic Syndrome

Traditionally, the thought was that people become obese, diabetic, insulin resistant, and so on through a diet with a high percentage of saturated fats.[35] But, recent studies indicate that a high intake of simple sugars common in soft drinks and refined carbohydrates also contribute to the alarming increase in metabolic syndrome.[36] To be more specific, the American Medical Association's (AMA) journal, *Circulation*, cited a study that nails soft drinks on the head. Participants who consumed one or more sodas daily prior to the study were 48 percent more likely to already have metabolic syndrome at the start of the study than those who consumed less. (It did not matter whether the participants consumed regular or diet soda.) Among those who did not begin the study with metabolic syndrome, participants who drank one or more sodas a day were 44 percent more likely to develop metabolic syndrome by the end of the study than those who drank less.[37]

The solution is simple: a better diet and more exercise. What constitutes a good diet depends on many things, but there seem to be a few common characteristics, like eating whole foods from green grocers and limiting your intake of foods that come out of containers, cardboard, cellophane, plastic, or any other man-made substance.[38] (For more detailed diet plans, see the Food Plans on page 111.)

It's a combination of both diet and exercise that will help you avoid metabolic syndrome. Research shows that higher intakes of fruit and vegetables are associated with a lower risk of metabolic syndrome and a lower C-reactive blood protein count. An elevated C-reactive protein count is one of the risk factors in metabolic syndrome, so the lower the better.[39]

So, eat your fruits and vegetables and get active. It will help you now, and in the long run.

DEMENTIA:
ROTTING TEETH, ROTTING BRAIN

Doctors and dentists agree that sugar rots teeth. However, there is less agreement on whether sugar causes heart disease, strokes, diabetes, and cancer. The thought that sugar may also cause mental impairment is even more controversial to the mainstream medical opinion.

Make no mistake—sugar can cause brain decay, more properly called dementia. Just when you thought you were safe with your statins for cholesterol, aspirin for your heart, and metabolizers for those excess pounds, dementia comes along, which means you might just be too forgetful to take your pills on time, causing a whole new array of problems. In the end, this could end up killing you faster then sugar alone.

What is Dementia?

Dementia is a decline in any mental function, including short- and long-term memory, logic, language, and personality. Most people think dementia only means Alzheimer's disease, which is the most common form of dementia, but there are other kinds. A stroke victim with a lot of impairment can be described as a dementia patient. So too can the unlucky who eat Mad Cow-infected beef. Mad Cow Disease is a fatal disease that cattle get. It affects the central nervous system, causing staggering and agitation in cows. In humans, the disease starts with confusion and personality and behavioral changes, and progresses to dementia. Most forms of dementia are thought of as older people's problems, as many think losing your mind is a natural part of growing older.

What Causes Dementia?

The science seems to indicate that sugar and dementia are closely related for the many forms of mental impairment you or your loved ones may suffer. Vascular dementia, the second most common form of dementia, seems to be common in people who have suffered strokes, hypertension (high blood pressure), or diabetes. It seems that there are two possible causes of vascular dementia. One is that sugar metabolism creates end products that directly attack nerve endings. The more widely accepted answer says that strokes, hypertension, and diabetes all serve to constrict blood flow to the brain, killing brain cells. If vascular dementia is highly associated with these sugar-related diseases, then it follows that the changes made to one's diet to deal with these other conditions would have a high likelihood of helping an ailing brain function at the same time.

Studies on Dementia

A four-year study on women with dementia found that about 6 percent of women with normal blood glucose levels developed or increased their symptoms of the disease. The same study concluded that the women with diabetes had a 12 percent increase of mental decline. There was also a third category that tested pre-diabetics who had an in-between condition called impaired fasting glucose, which is when glucose levels in the body are higher than normal in a fasting state, but not high enough to be diagnosed with diabetes. The pre-diabetics had a 10 percent increase of mental decline.[40]

A 1994 study dealing with insurance company Kaiser Permanente patients found results that linked dementia to obesity (another sugar-related ailment). The researchers dipped into the Health Maintenance Organization's (HMO) excellent records and surveyed people who, between 1964 and 1973, were between the ages of forty and forty-five and obese. The people were still patients in 1994 when the study was done. Those who were obese (a BMI of 30 or higher) were 74 percent more likely to contract some form of dementia in their later years, compared to those who had a normal BMI. Those classified as overweight (a BMI between 25 and 29.9) had a 35 percent greater risk of developing dementia. The study included both men and women.[41]

Other researchers approached the sugar and brain impairment relationship from other angles, like the C-Peptide marker. C-Peptide is an enzyme that is used as a marker on blood tests. C-Peptide marks how much insulin is in the bloodstream. If the C-Peptide is elevated on a blood test, it is highly indicative that the body is making more insulin than it needs because the muscles do not accept the insulin that is made and the pancreas keeps making more. The higher the C-peptide, the more insulin is in the bloodstream.

In one study, 718 women who were not diabetic gave blood samples, which indicated their C-Peptide levels. The study took place between June 14, 1989, and October 4, 1990, when the women were between the ages of sixty-one and sixty-nine (although the actual research wasn't done for another ten years). Telephone interviews were administered to the women in 2000 and then again two years later. The interviews questioned the participants to test for general cognition, verbal memory, and attention. The top 25 percent of the people with elevated C-Peptide levels in their blood tests were very likely to have developed a form of dementia a decade after giving blood. High levels of insulin in the blood can be detrimental to both diabetics and nondiabetics.[42]

In 2006, a Harvard Medical School researcher tested sixty patients over the age of seventy who had diabetes. The researcher used standardized tests for mental impairment on the patients. The study also included tests for depression. The test results showed that 33 percent of the subjects suffered from depression symptoms. According to the National Institute of Mental Health (NIMH), only 1 to 5 percent of non-diabetic elderly Americans suffer from depression. The results also showed that 38 percent of the test subjects scored low on the mental impairment test. It has been established that too much sugar in the diet can cause diabetes.

These test results show that 38 percent of all the diabetics tested had cognitive decline. In the general population, 22 percent of people have a cognitive decline by age seventy.[43]

Stopping Brain Decay

Science seems to indicate that sugar consumption and dementia are related.

While I can't help with Mad Cow Disease, I can help with most other forms of dementia, and that is with the same advice I give for your other problems: stop eating sugar, stop eating the foods you're allergic to, deal with your emotional and spiritual problems, and get some exercise. The research that I have shown certainly makes a case for removing sugar from your diet and dealing with depression. No one wants to walk around only half there in a depressed state, but your odds of doing so get greater with the more sugar you eat.

CANCER:
A CANCER ANSWER

No one wants to hear the word "cancer" spoken anywhere near them. Admit it, if you were at the doctor's office, you'd curl up into a ball and hope the doctor in the other room was speaking about another patient. Instinctively, we may think it's catching and we have to remind ourselves that it isn't contagious—at least not in the ordinary sense. But with the way we eat sugar and don't exercise, it might as well be.

Cancer is a word that describes the process of the body's cells growing out of control and the disease that results. Research shows that even in healthy people some cells are continuously being damaged and mutated by the various forms of natural stressors that exist in our environment, regardless of our diet and modern lifestyle. However, healthy people may never have to worry about getting cancer because their immune systems still work to eradicate all threats—usually before their next regularly scheduled doctor visit.

What Causes Cancer?

An unhealthy person may get cancer because he or she has suppressed his or her immune system with diet and distress. The cells that have been damaged by the environment will not have any checks and balances and will therefore continue to grow, so cancer may develop. Cancer, simply put, is a disease where damaged or abnormal cells of any type grow out of control.[44]

I have already made my general case that mineral imbalances caused by sugar and other dietary insults affect the proper functioning of hormones on which the immune and other body systems depend. When it comes to cancer, this immune suppression should be the first reason to completely avoid sugar during treatment. If the immune system heals and starts working, just imagine how much more effective many forms of cancer therapy will be.

People get cancer for different reasons. Some smoke too much. Some breathe in a lot of the polluted air in our cities. Some drink water that is either polluted or, in some cases, overly chlorinated. Other causes or risk factors for cancer may include sun exposure, viruses like the human papillomavirus (HPV), toxins, asbestos, food contamination, pesticides, and others.

Research has also shown that diets high in protein and low in vegetables, like many of the variations of the western diet, are linked to higher rates of cancer. Age is also a factor because the longer a body functions, the more likely something will happen to damage or mutate cells. Therefore, older people have a higher risk of developing cancer. Lastly, some people are just born with the genetic susceptibility for cancer, and if they lead a lifestyle that continually challenges their immune system, they will be more likely to develop cancer.

Sugar Feeds Cancer

Sugar has been linked to the cancer process ever since Dr. Otto Warburg won the 1931 Nobel Prize in Medicine for his work on cancer's energy cycle. He discovered that normal cells function best with oxygen as a catalyst for energy transfer, while abnormal cells transfer energy without oxygen. This oxygen-deficient cancer process is similar to how muscles create lactic acid after hard exercise, or how bacteria-like brewer's yeast converts sugars or plant fibers into alcohol, carbon dioxide, and water. All of these processes are sugar-dependent.

Warburg also described how a cancer causes the body to make sugars from proteins instead of carbohydrates or fat. This process, called glycogenesis, leads to the body wasting away because the body starves itself to feed the cancer. Additionally, the body must keep up with the expansion rate of the cancer cells, which is eight times faster than the expansion rate of normal cells. Eventually, more often than not, death results.[45]

There are other clues that sugar feeds cancer. It is no accident that positron emission tomography (PET) scans can be used to detect cancer by adding a slightly radioactive glucose solution to the bloodstream. The solution races directly to the cancer, and the radiation highlights abnormal areas of the brain and other tissues.[46] The various hospitals that perform PET scans explain on their websites that the brain, heart, and lungs consume copious amounts of sugar from the solution, leaving behind the radioactivity to measure any changes in these affected areas. But, the PET scan is also used to detect cancer anywhere in the body, so perhaps cancer consumes sugar like it were going out of style.[47]

Since the pancreas makes the insulin that helps us deal with the sugar in our bloodstream, this organ is a logical next step for exploring how sugar feeds cancer. Patients with pancreatic cancer have a survival rate of 4 percent in their fifth year after diagnosis. Approximately 30,000 Americans are diagnosed with pancreatic cancer every year.

An eighteen-year study followed 180 women who had pancreatic cancer. The researchers took note of the glycemic index (GI) of the foods the patients ate. To refresh, GI measures the rate at which an individual food raises blood sugar levels. Multiplying the GI by the total number of carbohydrates in the food and dividing that number by 100 yields the glycemic load (GL). (For more information on GI and GL, see page 29). The researchers cross-referenced the GI and GL with other factors in the patients' lives, including smoking, exercise levels, history of diabetes, fructose intake, and BMI. These were the results:

- Overweight women (having a BMI over 25) with inactive lifestyles who had high-GL diets (a GL over 20) were at the highest risk of pancreatic cancer.

- Women with active lifestyles who had high-GL diets were 53 percent more likely to develop pancreatic cancer than active women with low-GL diets.

- Women with active lifestyles and high fructose intake were 57 percent more likely to develop pancreatic cancer than active women who had low-GL diets.[48]

In North Carolina, a survey was conducted to determine which foods and beverages cancer patients preferred. A total of 222 adult oncology patients participated in the survey while in an oncology clinic for treatment or at a doctor's office for an appointment. Foods requested by at least 50 percent of the respondents included several types of crackers, doughnuts, fruit cups, cookies, applesauce, and gelatin cups. Beverages requested by at least 50 percent of the respondents included filtered water, coffee, soft drinks, and various juices.

Where is the whole food? The immune system of a cancer patient is supposed to be working on fighting the cancer, not on what the patient is eating. As we have seen, sugar feeds cancer. If only these people had the correct information.[49]

Other studies into the various types of cancer have shown the link between high sugar consumption and cancer. At least one included results correlating a high rate of type-2 diabetes with a similarly high rate of breast cancer in women.[50]

Studies show similar results from around the world. A lung cancer survey in Uruguay showed that people with high rates of smoking, fat intake, and sucrose consumption had significantly higher cancer risks over people with healthier habits in those areas. The risk for sucrose by itself was still moderately high.[51]

The same researchers expanded their study to include colon cancer, finding that high sucrose intake resulted in a slightly more than doubled risk of developing colon cancer. Glucose produced a risk slightly less than sucrose. They also found an interesting link between sucrose and high levels of protein intake. This risk was close to five times that of sucrose or glucose alone.[52]

Sugar not only helps cancer get started, it also accelerates cancer growth. A mouse study of human breast cancer demonstrated that tumors are sensitive to blood glucose levels. Sixty-eight mice were injected with an aggressive strain of breast cancer and then fed diets to induce either high blood sugar (hyperglycemia), normal blood sugar (normoglycemia), or low blood sugar (hypoglycemia). There was a dose-dependent response that showed the lower the blood glucose, the greater the survival rate. After seventy days, nineteen out of twenty hypoglycemic mice survived compared to sixteen out of twenty-four normoglycemic mice and eight out of twenty-four hyperglycemic mice. The authors of the study suggest that regulating sugar intake is key to slowing breast tumor growth. I, however, think the results of the study speak loud and clear—cancer patients shouldn't just regulate sugar intake. A cancer patient should eat no sugar at all, nor should he or she eat any fruit or drink any fruit juice.[53]

Let me point out here that while sugar is a primary culprit in getting and succumbing to cancer, a patient's mental state has almost as much effect on cancer as their diet. Researchers found that people without cancer who experienced an event that triggered long-term depression and hopelessness lasting at least a year had increased rates of cancer within the next three years. The study went on to conclude that momentary anger or other negative emotions had almost no effect on cancer rates, suggesting that long-term unrequited negativity is the problem.[54]

Avoiding Cancer

Cancer can be fought with diet and a positive outlook. If you are diagnosed with cancer, you should cut all sugar out of your diet, including fruit, in order to starve the tumor of all sugars. Whole fruit may be good for healthy people, but even the naturally-occurring sugar in whole fruit can feed a tumor.

Food Plan III (see page 112) includes removal of all possible sources of dietary sugar: sweets, fruit, and most importantly, soft drinks. This will help starve the tumor of its food, which should allow the cancer treatment to work more effectively. Sugar feeds cancer and getting and keeping the fasting blood glucose down below 100 mg/dL will help with cancer and many other diseases. Food Plan III is designed to do this.

You should also remember to ask for all your results when you have laboratory work done in a doctor's office. You are in charge of your health. You will get back blood tests with the levels of blood glucose that you can compare from time to time, as well as many other factors to use for comparison. You can also give your tests to another doctor to view.

This book is mainly about sugar, but stressful situations can also play a role in cancer (as noted by the study discussed previously). You could sit down to the perfect meal but if you are angry or have other negative emotions, the food may not be digested well. Toxicity can occur and can lead to cancer and other diseases developing. It is not life's situations, but how we deal with them that matters. Resolving those emotions through therapy, groups, writing in journals, exercise, prayer, or a combination of all will certainly help you in the long run. It is amazing how we create so many illnesses ourselves, but we can also recreate our lives for health.

EPILEPSY: SWEET SEIZURE

My research on sugar end products attacking nerve cells is logically applicable to epilepsy and seizures, as well.

What is Epilepsy?

According to *Mosby's Medical, Nursing, & Allied Health Dictionary*, epilepsy is a recurrent episode of convulsive seizures, sensory disturbances, abnormal behavior, loss of consciousness, or a combination of all of these. The seizures can occur many times a day or not for years.

Faraway Places

The health effects of sugar are not exclusive to the western world. From the Amazon River communities to the villages in China, western food has made its debut and mark on the whole world.

One of my greatest pleasures is to travel to parts of the world that few other Americans can even find on the map. I typically come back with stories about what I did and where I went, and I bring back gifts for my children. I also scoop up all the native fabrics I can find.

My children have come to expect the stories and fabrics, especially the ones with bright colors. And then, since they have more or less been with me from the beginning of my journey to better health, the conversation eventually gets around to how the people in these underdeveloped places eat. I regret to report that sugar has invaded there as well as here—the only difference being to what degree.

The Influence of the West

The degenerative diseases that have scourged the developed world since sugar's introduction are encroaching on the diet of the developing world. Coca-Cola is everywhere. It is said that Coca-Cola, Elvis, and Jesus are three of the most recognizable symbols in the world. American marketing is responsible for Coca-Cola, Elvis, and possibly Jesus reaching that status.

When I see neon signs for Burger King in downtown Beijing, I wonder when Chinese health authorities will make the connection that the western diet is changing their country for the worse. I have been to hospitals in the capital of Papua New Guinea where death rates from heart disease, cancer, and diabetes are similar to ours. I have also been able to go to the rural hospitals in Papua New Guinea where few people have these diseases. I try to tell doctors in developing countries to put their patients back on the native diet wherever possible, but I get the same shrugs of acceptance and frustration wherever I go.

We typically think of the developing world as places where infectious diseases (such as malaria, tuberculosis, and pneumonia) still afflict people. The modern world zapped these diseases with antibiotics long ago in the big cities, although these infectious diseases still plague the villages around the world. However, sugar is very addictive—this goes for all countries, but double for any part of the world that may be lacking in essential knowledge. Of course, to say the developed world has much more knowledge about diet, exercise, and sugar may stretch the point. But, at least we have a few doctors here who know to tell their patients to walk more and eat more fruits and vegetables. Unfortunately, even here very few doctors tell their patients to cut out sugar.

The Effect on the Developing World

One of my main points in this book is that sugar and processed, over-cooked foods (courtesy of the western diet) wreak havoc on the immune system, which defends against infectious and certain degenerative diseases. Therefore, if a native of a region lacking basic sanitation and refrigeration drinks a Coca-Cola or eats a candy bar, he or she will be prone to more infectious or degenerative diseases. The immune system can only take so many insults and then it becomes exhausted. Lack of sanitation and refrigeration and a dose of sugar can make the body a target for diseases.

I'm not the only one noticing this change in diets around the world. On November 16, 1995, I was in my hotel room in Trier, Germany watching CNN. Imagine my surprise to see a story from Mexico about the effect the modern diet has on prenatal care and childhood development.

The report showed pictures of obese pregnant women sucking on long, plastic tubes of colored sugar ice, much like a Slurpee. With these mothers were some of their children. The reporter told the audience that a local study confirmed that the intellectual performance of the kids born to those women would likely never reach their full potential because of the diet of the mothers. I nearly danced in front of the TV.

The report went on to say that those kids were considered malnourished because they weren't getting the nutrients present in a regular diet, which are essential to cognitive function. Since this has been one of my main points all along, you will understand how I enjoyed having a key piece of my program acknowledged. The reporter said that the parents could not afford to buy rice and beans, and that the sugar water filled them up. I do not agree with that conclusion. I believe the women were addicted to sugar and could not quit.

A week later, CNN surprised me again by reporting another health story, this time from Rio de Janeiro. Essentially, the story covered the change from farmers growing corn to farmers growing wheat. In one bakery, 30,000 wheat buns were sold on the day CNN taped the report.

Wheat is easier than corn to process into precooked items, which free the women of Rio de Janeiro from some kitchen tasks. Most of these precooked foods are made from white flour, which is wheat that has been bleached to look more appealing. However, the process of bleaching wheat essentially strips it of the vitamins and nutrients that made it healthy to our ancestors. I've always suspected that the white sugar added to the "Staff of Life" (wheat) hastened its change into a food that should be avoided.

Additionally, corn cannot be made into bread or baked goods by itself. It needs the gluten from wheat to make it stick together. Therefore, it is difficult to make cookies, pastries, cakes, pies, and other sugary goodies out of corn—but not out of wheat. Now that the people in these developing countries are able to bake sugary treats, they will be getting lots of refined carbohydrates from wheat that they do not need. Baked white flour is more difficult to digest than boiled wheat.

The World Bank, an organization that provides assistance to developing countries around the world, is firmly behind the process of wheat replacement around the world, since their main concern is that undernourished countries eat something; anything.

The Irony of it All

What's ironic is that in my travels, the native diet has always been superior for health. In China, the native diet is fish, chicken, and rice. Many Chinese natives also spend their days either working in the fields or riding bikes to work in the cities. This exercise helps. In Africa, the diet is rice, beans, meat, and whatever vegetables grow naturally. In many places, the countryside does better than the city because in the country, the western diet only makes a sporadic appearance.

It's also ironic that the native diet is cheaper for most people to afford. Beans and rice come in at pennies per pound almost everywhere I've gone. The problem is that sugar is addictive, and therefore, some people will spend the extra money in order to feed their cravings. Some natives even acknowledge the fact that there is a sugar problem in their country, and also that they simply don't know what to do to fix it. I've sat across from plenty of local healers who tell me how much wheat and sugar is in the diets of locals. They all seem to have the same smile, and they appreciate my knowledge and research. But there is still that slight nod that tells me, "Excellent idea, Dr. Appleton. But when you find out how to convince more than a few people at a time, please call me."

Meanwhile, I long to hear the call of another place I have yet to see, where the fabrics are bright and the diet is something like what early man ate. Although I have eaten this diet in villages across the world, these foods are more difficult to obtain each year, thanks to sugar, white, processed flour, McDonalds, Jack in the Box, and Coca-Cola.

Studies on Epilepsy

One clue to sugar's influence on seizures comes from a rat study. The researchers added sucrose to the diets of female rats who were on lithium and pilocarpine, drugs used to induce a seizure. They measured the time between subsequent seizures, which came more frequently with the addition of sugar. I'll let the researchers' conclusion of the study speak for itself—the findings suggest that a diet supplemented with sugar can facilitate the emergence of behavioral seizures in female rats given lithium and pilocarpine.[55] We've already discussed how the results of mouse and rat studies can parallel the results a similar study would likely have on humans.

Preventing Epilepsy

The Epilepsy Foundation endorses a ketogenic diet to help keep the issue under control.[56]

A ketogenic diet is a diet of mostly fat and protein with some vegetables. Absolutely no sugar is allowed for people on this diet. A person on this diet cannot even take a medicine with sugar in it. A medical professional must regulate the ketogenic diet. I do not recommend this diet for a person suffering from epilepsy without the advice and consent of someone in the medical field. If you think this diet is right for you and your doctor won't recommend it, seek out another doctor.

The ketogenic diet is usually called for when traditional anticonvulsants have not been effective. To me, the logical solution would be to try this diet first so as not to invade the body with medications. Use medication only as a last resort. The fact that a person on this diet cannot eat any sugar tells me that sugar definitely plays a role somewhere in the epilepsy disease.

Mainstream doctors are very sure that mental impairment is permanent. This means that you have to do something now while you can still do things like read this book and comprehend information. It doesn't matter whether your mind goes because of vascular constriction (a classic stroke) or if too much insulin impedes mental function—once it's gone, it's gone.

When we continually upset our body's chemistry, we are more likely to get the disease of our family's choice. If there are people in your family that have cancer, you could have a genetic blueprint for cancer. You might also have a genetic blueprint for heart disease or any other disease. If we do not continually upset our body chemistry we do not have to manifest those diseases. Some people eat sugar and junk food, ignore their allergies, and hide from their emotional life. Some get heart attacks, some get cancer, and others slowly lose their minds. I think the research in this section proves the point that you could be causing your own brain to rot, and sugar can play a significant role in that.

CONCLUSION

Unfortunately, this is just the tip of the iceberg. Since many people have the symptoms and diseases discussed, I hope that the information in this chapter will help you understand why added sugar plays such a devastating role in many degenerative disease processes. Of course, when sugar suppresses your immune system, you open the door to all infectious diseases also.

So, what now? You've got all the information about sugar under your belt. The question is, what are you going to do with it? You have two options: either ignore everything you've learned and continue to damage your body, or take the information at hand and choose to do something about it. It's never too late to change your life for the better.

The following chapter contains information about cutting sugar out of your diet in order to live an all-around healthier lifestyle. Make the wise decision—turn the page and start living healthier.

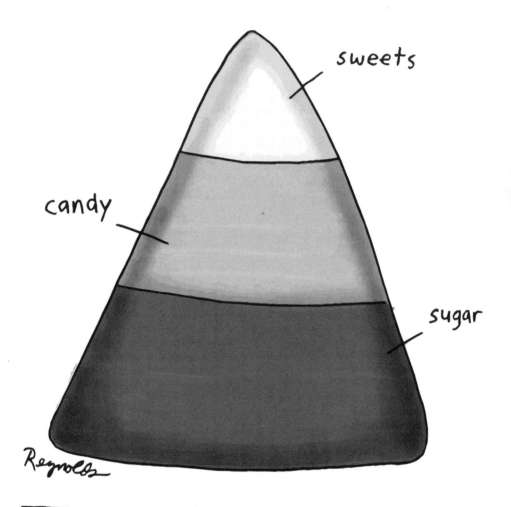

7

A Practical Plan
for Right Now

We are in a time of incredible technological advances and material abundance, and yet the money we spend on healthcare is not getting us better healthcare. Read on about this dichotomy of money and medical research verses wellness and healthcare.

In 2005, total national health expenditures rose 6.9 percent from 2004—two times the rate of inflation. Total spending was $2 trillion in 2005, or roughly $6,700 per person. Total healthcare spending represented 16 percent of the gross domestic product (GDP).[1] Healthcare spending in the United States is expected to keep increasing at similar levels, reaching $4 trillion in 2015, or 20 percent of the GDP.[2]

Healthcare spending in the United States is 4.3 times the amount spent on national defense. Although nearly 47 million Americans are uninsured, the United States spends more on healthcare than other industrialized nations do—and those countries provide health insurance to all their citizens.[3]

Healthcare spending accounted for 10.9 percent of the GDP in Switzerland, 10.7 percent in Germany, 9.7 percent in Canada, and 9.5 percent in France, according to the Organization for Economic Cooperation and Development.[4] So, those are the monetary statistics about healthcare. It is scary information.

It doesn't get better when you read about life expectancy and infant mortality. In 2006, records of the nations with the largest populations showed that the Japanese live the longest with a life expectancy of 82.2 years. After Japan came many countries, including Singapore, Hong Kong, Australia, New Zealand, Israel, and

Canada. The United States hit the list at Number 45 with a life expectancy of 78 years.[5]

To continue this dreary tale, infant mortality rates are not any better. Singapore has the lowest rate of infant mortality, with only 2.3 deaths per 1,000 live births in 2006. The same countries that live the longest are ahead of us on these statistics. But there are a few other countries whose infant mortality is less than ours that you might not have guessed. They are Slovenia, South Korea, and Cuba. It is almost embarrassing to think that those countries lose less babies than we do in childbirth with all our spending, educated doctors, and research. The United States came in at Number 41 with 6.4 deaths per 1,000 live births. It seems to me we must be doing something wrong.[6]

You may be interested in finding out what the fattest countries in the world are. The fattest is Nauru, one of the smallest countries in the world, an 8-square mile coral island, lying just south of the equator near Papua New Guinea. It is a very wealthy island because of its phosphate resources. Of course, wealth brings sugar and junk food. Most of the other nations with citizens who weigh more than United States citizens are small islands and Kuwait. The United States weighs in with 74.1 percent of the population being overweight. The United States is Number 9 on a list of twenty of the fattest countries in the world. These statistics are based on people age fifteen and older. The only other developed nation on the list is Argentina—there are no European countries on the list. People are considered overweight if their BMI is between 25 and 29.9, and they are considered obese if their BMI is 30 or higher.[7] (For more on BMI, see page 44.)

I believe that these statistics have a lot to do with sugar, which is why I included them. Sugar is the main problem, but the rest of our eating patterns and lifestyle factors also play a role.

These health statistics are not complimentary at all to the United States. You read earlier that we eat a lot of sugar, about 142 pounds of sugar per person per year. The U.S. government subsidizes sugar to the tune of about $2 billion annually.[8] In essence, we are all helping to pay for these problems. In Chapter 2, you learned about 140 problems that sugar can cause (see page 13). This makes a good case for the effects of sugar on our health and on our pocketbook. It seems quite evident to me that this substance should be removed as much as possible from our diets.

Dr. Linus Pauling, a Nobel Prize winner in chemistry and a researcher and writer in the health field, once said, "If I had to remove one food from my diet, it would be sugar." Good idea, Dr. Pauling.

BREAKING THE SUGAR ADDICTION

There are numerous ways to break an addiction. The most common, going cold turkey, is a losing proposition. The withdrawal symptoms can be overwhelming and drive the sufferer back to sugar to ease his or her stressed body.

It's better to ease out of the addiction. Try dividing your sugar from all sources in half. This means half as much sugar in your coffee, tea, or lemonade. For foods where the sugar comes premixed or baked in, don't buy them. Try making your own food. Do this for one week.

The second week, try limiting yourself to just one bite of the sweet food you want to eat, then push the plate away. Many years ago, when I wanted to help my kids stop eating sugar, I started off by limiting them to one dessert per day. I used the progression listed above until I eliminated sugar from the house. Sure, they snuck sugar back into their diets out of the house, but I made sure my kids ate at least two meals a day in the house, so I still felt I was ahead of the game.

It's important to remember that emotional well-being also affects health. Blaming yourself for your cravings will not help the problem. Being sad or depressed can lead to low levels of serotonin or other neurotransmitters, which can also cause cravings. Therefore, getting angry at yourself for being unable to resist a craving may in turn cause future cravings.

Some addictions are so strong that they can not be conquered by using willpower and resistance techniques. In these situations, a twelve-step program can help. They meet pretty much anywhere civilized. Two groups that have twelve-step programs that can be particularly helpful to sugar addicts are Food Addicts in Recovery (FA) and Food Addicts Anonymous (FAA). (For more information on these groups, see Resources on page 143.) I have been to a few meetings and I've seen that these groups offer long-term help for sugar addicts.

As Mark Twain said of his cigars, "Quitting is easy. I have done it many times." I have quit sugar more times than I would have liked.

But, I did not know as much as you do about what sugar was doing to me. Also, there were no support groups, as there are today, to help me along the way.

TIPS FOR HEALTHY LIVING

I want to provide a few suggestions because I believe that much of the damage from sugar can be reversed. I spend so much time on sugar because it is the obvious culprit in our society. There are other ways to upset your body chemistry—mental, emotional, physical, environmental, and so forth—but I always come back to diet and sugar, because of the massive damage they do to our society.

Most people need to work on their sugar habit first. After licking the sugar habit, if you understand the following principles, they will form a solid foundation for maintaining good health:

- After a health breakdown, the way in which your body responds to appropriate medical care depends on your body chemistry's ability to rebalance.

- Body chemistry may become unbalanced quickly. Depending on an individual's adaptive abilities, body chemistry may stay unbalanced or rebalance just as quickly.

- Both disease and good health are the result of the condition of the body's chemistry. Health breakdowns result from an unbalanced body chemistry, which results from minerals being out of their proper relationships.

- The extent of any health breakdown is determined by the degree and duration of the chemical imbalance.

- The only difference between a healthy person and a sick person is that the healthy person's body can efficiently rebalance his or her body chemistry.

- Through conscious and unconscious choices, you can control your body's chemical balance.

Understanding and acting upon these principles will help you regain and maintain good health.

Everyone is unique and each person responds differently to various therapies. For some, simple lifestyle modifications can greatly improve health. Others need more help searching for the right methods to help their bodies heal.

HOMEOSTASIS TESTING

Another aspect of getting and staying healthy is determining which foods are most likely to upset your individual body chemistry. The Body Monitor Kit can help you discover what those foods are. It can also show how well you maintain your health. You will learn which foods are digesting properly and if the stress in your life is becoming distress and upsetting your body.

The test works by measuring the amount of calcium in the urine. It lets you know if you are secreting too much, too little, or a normal amount of calcium. Calcium only works in relation to phosphorus, so no calcium in the urine means that too much phosphorus is present and too much calcium in the urine means not enough phosphorus is present. A normal result means the minerals are likely in balance.

While the test checks only for calcium, it is a safe assumption that any abnormal result means that all minerals are out of balance. A normal calcium result means that the body is in homeostasis and the vitamins, minerals, and enzymes all work properly.

The kit comes with instructions that explain its use (see page 182 for ordering information).

FOOD PLANS

The following food plans are effective in helping your body achieve and maintain homeostasis. You might start by continuing to eat the meals and snacks that you have been eating, and then using the Body Monitor Kit to see if your body is in homeostasis. If you are in homeostasis before and after you eat your food, you know that the meals are digesting and metabolizing correctly. If you do not see homeostasis, I suggest you start on Food Plan I and see if that gets you back to homeostasis. If not, go on to Food Plan II and, if necessary, III. The booklet that comes with the kit, *How to Monitor Your Basic Health*, is far more detailed and gives you specific suggestions. Those of you who don't have the kit should still follow the food plans. Even if you don't test to see if your body is in homeostasis, you will still be eating healthy and likely feeling better than you have in a long time.

If you experience symptoms such as headaches, joint pains, general fatigue (especially after meals), and high blood pressure, or if you have a degenerative disease, you might start out following Food Plan III. If after a week you still cannot regain and maintain homeostasis, I suggest that you do a green juice diet for two days and then try testing again. You can get green juices at health food stores or you can make them yourself with a juicer. You can use celery, carrots, spinach, kale, or any green vegetable and mix it with a little carrot juice. Drink about $1^1/_2$ quarts of the juice a day, and also drink fresh water.

Be aware that in following the food plans, you may experience withdrawal symptoms caused by eliminating the addictive foods from your diet. These symptoms can include fever, depression, headaches, chills, anger, and fatigue. For some people, these symptoms may last two or three days, but others may feel them for up to a week.

All the food plans refer to foods from the different category lists beginning on page 114, which follow the food plans. Be sure to refer to these lists.

Food Plan I

- Avoid all foods and substances from Categories IV and V. Eat all other foods.

- Remain on this diet for seven days and evaluate your symptoms or your urine tests. A lack of results means your body chemistry may require a more stringent food plan. If this is the case, you may need to try Food Plan II.

Food Plan II

- Avoid all foods from Categories III, IV, and V. Eat only foods from Category I and Category II.

- Remain on this diet for seven days and evaluate your symptoms or your urine tests. Poor results suggest it may be time for Food Plan III.

Food Plan III

If you're considering this plan, your unbalanced body needs some serious help to find foods you won't react to. This plan is designed to provide the body with complete nutrients in their best form. Most people can digest, metabolize, and assimilate the foods on this plan easily. The procedures and foods here are the least stressful to your body chemistry.

- For fourteen days, eat only foods from Category I. Eat one small portion from each food group four or five times a day.

- Follow the Healthy Eating Habits later in this chapter, beginning on page 118.

- If after fourteen days you are still not experiencing symptom relief, you likely need professional help. Seek out a qualified practitioner who can test your blood for food sensitivities. You are still reacting to foods that upset your body chemistry.

Simple Suggestions for Breakfast and Snacks

People who are on Food Plan III sometimes run into trouble with breakfast. Before I became healthy, I ate chocolate cake for breakfast. Now my thought pattern goes like this: if I could eat chocolate cake for breakfast many years ago, why can't I eat vegetables for breakfast now? Neither of these foods fit into the usual breakfast eating pattern. I am now hooked on vegetables for breakfast. Here are some suggestions you can try:

- Baked potato with butter, guacamole, or pureed beans.

- Cooked potatoes, refrigerated overnight, sliced and sautéed in butter.

- Cooked rice with butter.

- Corn tortilla with butter, tomatoes, scrambled egg and/or guacamole.

- Cream of rice with butter.

- Leftover rice with grated carrots, grated onions, peas, lima beans and butter (my favorite).

- Oatmeal with butter (not instant oatmeal).

- One cup of popped corn with butter.

- One-egg omelet with sliced and diced tomato and vegetables.

- One-egg Ranchero with corn tortilla (see page 120 for recipe).

- Rice cakes with sliced avocado, tomato, onion, green pepper, or cucumber.

- Steamed sweet potato with butter (also good cold).

Food Categories

Vegetarians and vegans may eliminate foods from the fish and meat/poultry lists as they please. If you are a vegetarian or vegan, you should remember to eat more beans and grains for complete protein. If you follow your metabolic type or if you eat according to your blood type, you can also use these food plans very easily. In fact, it does not matter what type of diet you are on or not on, you can still use these food plans.

Category I

When properly prepared and eaten, people with unbalanced body chemistry best tolerate the following foods. Remove any reactive foods (foods to which you react negatively to, or foods to which you are allergic).

Green Leafy Vegetables

Artichoke	Cabbage	Lettuce (all)
Brussels sprouts	Kale	Spinach

Green Vegetables

Alfalfa	Broccoli	Chinese pea pods
Asparagus	Celery	Okra
Avocado		

Root Vegetables

Jicama	Potato	Rutabaga
Onion	Radish	Turnip
Parsnip		

Yellow/White Vegetables

Cauliflower	Cucumber	Squash (all)
Corn		

Orange/Purple/Red Vegetables

Beet	Eggplant	Sweet potato
Carrot	Pumpkin	Tomato

Herbs/Condiments

Arrowroot	Garlic	Parsley
Basil	Ginger	Rose hips
Bay leaf	Horseradish	Rosemary
Black pepper	Lemon	Safflower oil
Butter	Lime	Sage
Caraway	Mustard	Sesame oil
Chili pepper	Nutmeg	Sunflower oil
Chive	Olive oil	Tarragon
Cilantro	Oregano	Thyme
Dill		

Fish

Anchovy	Halibut	Shark
Bass	Mackerel	Shrimp
Catfish	Oyster	Sole
Clam	Perch	Swordfish
Cod	Red snapper	Trout
Crab	Salmon	Tuna
Flounder	Sardine	Any other fish
Haddock	Scallop	

Meats/Poultry

Bacon	Duck	Pork
Beef	Lamb	Turkey
Chicken	Liver (beef/chicken)	Venison
Eggs	Pheasant	

Beans/Grains

Azuki beans	Kidney beans	Red beans
Barley	Lentils	Rice, brown
Bean sprouts	Lima beans	Rice, white
Black beans	Millet	Rice, wild
Black-eyed peas	Navy beans	Rye
Buckwheat	Oats	Soybeans
Garbanzo beans	Pinto beans	Split peas
Green beans	Quinoa	White beans
Green peas		

Category II

Some body chemistries are sensitive to these otherwise wholesome foods.

Fruits

Apples	Figs	Peaches
Apricots	Grapes	Pears
Bananas	Guava	Pineapples
Cantaloupe	Melons (all)	Raspberries
Coconuts	Nectarines	Strawberries
Cranberries	Papayas	Watermelon
Dates		

Nuts/Seeds

Almonds	Macadamia nuts	Sesame seeds
Brazil nuts	Pecans	Sunflower seeds
Chestnuts	Pistachios	Tahini
Hazelnuts	Poppy seeds	Walnuts
Hickory nuts	Safflower seeds	

Herbs/Condiments

Anise seeds	Clove	Paprika
Chicory	Cream of tartar	Spearmint

Category III

Overcooking, overeating, and eating foods with sugar have turned these normally well-tolerated foods into potentially abusive ones in some people, including those who have already compromised their systems through continued abuse.

Grains

Kamut	Wheat bran	Wheat germ
Rye	Whole wheat	White flour
Spelt		

Dairy

Buttermilk	Cream cheese	Whey
Cheese (all)	Milk, cow's	Yogurt

Fungi

Mushrooms	Yeast, baker's	Yeast, brewer's

Fruits

Grapefruit	Orange	Tangerine
Mango		

Nuts/Seeds

Cashews	Peanuts

Miscellaneous

Carob	Cornstarch	Salt
Cinnamon	Curry	Tea, decaf
Coffee, decaf	Hops	Tea, regular
Coffee, regular	Molasses	Vanilla
Cola bean	Peppermint	

Category IV

These foods are generally reactive to everyone. Only those with adaptive abilities remaining will rebalance after frequent exposure to these foods. The more Category IV foods you consume, the more rapid the deteriorations in your body chemistry will occur.

Alcohol	Corn sugar	Maple sugar
Barley malt	Corn syrup	Rice syrup
Beet sugar	Fructose	Saccharin
Cane sugar	Honey	All other forms of sugar
Cocoa	Malt	

Category V

The items on this list are substances with similar effects to Category IV, but with even less nutritional value. There are drugs, preservatives, fillers, and coloring agents found in processed foods on this list. Use them sparingly or, better yet, not at all. Read your labels!

Acetaminophen	Food coloring	Petroleum byproducts
Aspirin	Formaldehyde	Sodium benzoate
Butylated hydroxotoluene	Ibuprofen	Soft drinks
Drugs (all)*	Monosodium glutamate	Sports drinks
Energy drinks		Tobacco

Over-the-counter, prescription, street

HEALTHY EATING HABITS

Regardless of which food plan you follow, be sure to observe the following healthy eating habits.

- Ask yourself, "Will this affect my body chemistry?"

- Chew each bite twenty times.

- Consume portions that are digestible to you.

- Don't overcook your food.

- Don't wash food down with liquids—swallow, then drink.

- If emotionally upset or disturbed, eat smaller portions and chew longer—better yet, wait to eat.

- Instead of big meals less often, eat small meals more often.

- Split your plate evenly between cooked and raw foods.

Eating small portions of many foods is better than having a large portion of a single food. Following these eating habits will lessen body chemistry imbalances and facilitate more efficient digestion and usage of nutrients. Additionally, you will support your body's ability to rebalance, and your response to appropriate medical care will be improved.

RECIPES TO TAME YOUR SWEET TOOTH

All of the recipes in this book can be used with Food Plan III, the strictest diet. They do not contain sugar of any kind, nor do they contain fruit, fruit juice, nuts, seeds, wheat, or dairy—except butter and whipping cream. The problem with dairy products is that they contain lactose, to which many people have an adverse reaction. There is very little lactose in butter and whipping cream.

Instead of using regular butter in the recipes, you can also use clarified butter or ghee, which does not contain *any* milk. You can buy ghee or make your own, which is very simple. Slowly simmer butter in a pan for five minutes or so until a frothy foam (the milk solids) forms on top. Remove the pan from the heat and let cool. Skim the foam from the top. What's left is ghee.

If you want to use a sweetener in some of these recipes, I recommend Stevia, a non-caloric natural sweetener that comes in liquid, powder, and pill form. (Make sure you do not use any of the sugars on page 10.) I find liquid Stevia the easiest for controlling added sweetness to foods and beverages. However, I believe that each person is different, and it is best to use whichever form of Stevia works best for you. Stevia is available at health food stores and many larger grocery stores.

EGGS RANCHEROS

(Found in breakfast suggestions for Food Plan III, page 113)

YIELD: 1 SERVING

1 corn tortilla

2 teaspoons butter

1 egg

Avocado slices for garnish

1. Poach the egg.

2. While the egg is cooking, melt the butter in a frying pan over medium heat. Add the tortilla and cook about a minute on each side.

3. Place the tortilla on a plate, add the poached egg, and top with heated salsa (see recipe below). Garnish with avocado slices and serve.

SALSA

Delicious salsa is an important component of eggs Rancheros. This salsa recipe makes about $2\frac{1}{2}$ cups (enough for four to five servings). Use what you need and store the rest in the refrigerator, where it will keep for at least a week.

16-ounce can tomatoes with juice

2 jalapeño peppers (or to taste)

$\frac{1}{4}$ teaspoon salt

$\frac{1}{4}$ teaspoon minced garlic

1 teaspoon olive oil

$\frac{1}{2}$ cup finely diced onion

2 tablespoons chopped fresh cilantro

1. To make the salsa, place the tomatoes, peppers, salt, garlic, and oil in a blender and pulse until well-blended but slightly chunky. Transfer to a bowl and stir in the onions and cilantro.

2. Salsa can be served warm or cold. (For eggs Rancheros recipe above, warm up $\frac{1}{2}$ cup of the salsa and pour over eggs Rancheros.)

SQUASH TART

YIELD: 4 SERVINGS

6 cups coarsely grated winter squash
(kobacha, delicata, butternut, etc.), loosely packed

$1/2$ teaspoon powdered ginger

$1/4$ teaspoon powdered cinnamon

$1/4$ teaspoon powdered coriander

$1/4$ teaspoon powdered cardamom

$1/2$ stick butter, softened

4 rice tortillas* (about 9 inches)

* Available in many health food stores

1. Preheat the oven to 350°F.

2. Place the squash, ginger, cinnamon, coriander, and cardamom in a bowl and stir to mix well.

3. Place one of the tortillas in a buttered 9-inch pie pan and top with 2 cups of the squash mixture. Place another tortilla on top, brush with butter, and repeat the layers, ending with the last tortilla on top.

4. Brush the top tortilla with butter and cover with parchment paper or aluminum foil.

5. Bake at 350°F for 30 minutes, then uncover and bake another 30 minutes, or until the top is golden brown and crisp.

6. Cut the tart in quarters and serve as is or topped with whipped cream.

Adapted recipe from Mil Kregu; Tierra Miguel Foundation (Tierramiguelfarm.org).

SWEET POTATO PANCAKES

YIELD: APPROXIMATELY 16 TO 20 PANCAKES

1 large sweet potato or yam, grated

1 large russet potato (about same size as the sweet potato), grated

1 medium onion, minced

1 small carrot, grated

2 eggs, slightly beaten

2 tablespoons rice flour

Freshly ground black pepper (to taste)

Freshly grated nutmeg (to taste)

$1/4$ cup sesame, coconut, or olive oil

1. Combine the grated potatoes, onions, and carrots in a colander and let drain for an hour. Transfer to a mixing bowl, add all of the remaining ingredients except the oil, and mix well. If the batter is too watery, add more rice flour.

2. Heat the oil in a large skillet over medium heat. Add $1/4$-cup amounts of the mixture to the hot skillet. Cook until the bottoms are brown, then turn and cook to brown the other side.

3. Enjoy the pancakes hot, warm, or at room temperature.

Adapted recipe from *Dr. Jo's Natural Healing Cookbook* by Bessie Jo Tillman, MD (www.dr-jo-md.com).

BAKED BEETS

YIELD: 4 SERVINGS

4 medium or 2 large beets

$1/2$ cup whipped cream

1. Preheat the oven to 375°F.

2. Scrub the beets with the skin on, then place in a baking dish. (If using large beets, cut them in half.) Bake for 45 minutes, or until tender. Remove and let cool until warm enough to handle.

3. Grate the beets on the large holes of a grater (the skin will not go through the holes).

4. Place equal amounts of the grated beets in four sherbet or parfait glasses. Top with whipped cream and serve.

Variation: Instead of whipped cream, try spooning heavy cream over the beets.

Adapted recipe from *The Candida Albicans Yeast-Free Cookbook* by Pat Connolly & Associates of the Price-Pottenger Nutrition Foundation (www.ppnf.org).

ZOILA'S SWEET POTATO MILLET MUFFINS

YIELD: 6 MUFFINS

1 cup well-mashed sweet potatoes

$1/2$ cup light olive or safflower oil

1 cup millet flour

1 teaspoon cinnamon

$1/8$ teaspoon sea salt

Dash baking soda

1. Preheat the oven to 350°F.

2. Place the potatoes and oil in a mixing bowl and stir until well-combined.

3. In a separate bowl, combine the flour, cinnamon, salt, and baking soda. Add to the potato mixture and stir to form a smooth batter. If batter is too thick, add unsweetened rice milk—a tablespoon at a time—until the consistency is smooth.

4. Ladle the batter into a greased 6-cup standard muffin pan. Bake for 50 to 60 minutes, or until a toothpick inserted in the center of a muffin comes out clean.

5. Cool the muffins about 10 minutes before removing from the tin. Serve warm or at room temperature.

Adapted recipe from Natasha Zarrin, graduate of the Natural Gourmet Institute, NYC (www.naturalgourmetschool.com).

RICH CAROB-AVOCADO MOUSSE

YIELD: 2 SERVINGS

1 ripe avocado, peeled and pitted

6 teaspoons carob powder

2 tablespoons heavy whipping cream

$1/2$ teaspoon vanilla extract

1. Combine all of the ingredients in a food processor and blend at high speed until smooth. For lighter texture, add more whipping cream 1 teaspoon at a time until the desired texture is reached.

2. Spoon the mousse into two parfait glasses and serve.

Adapted recipe from Mil Kregu; Tierra Miguel Foundation (Tierramiguelfarm.org).

CARROT PUFF

YIELD: 4 SERVINGS

2 cups finely diced carrots

2 tablespoons butter

1 cup minced onions

1 egg, separated

$1/4$ teaspoon salt

Generous dash ground cloves

4 lemon wedges

1. Preheat the oven to 350°F. Butter a 9-x-5-inch loaf pan and set aside.

2. Steam the carrots about 20 minutes, or until very tender.

3. Melt the butter in a small frying pan over medium-low heat. Add the onions, and cook about 5 minutes, or until tender.

4. Place the carrots and onions to a blender and purée. You can also use a potato ricer for this.

5. Transfer the carrot-onion mixer to a bowl along with the egg yolk, salt, and cloves, and beat until smooth. In a separate bowl, beat the

egg white with an electric mixer until stiff peaks form. Fold the egg white into the carrot mixture.

6. Turn the mixture into the prepared loaf pan and bake for 20 to 25 minutes, or until a toothpick inserted in the center comes out clean.

7. Scoop out portions of the hot "puff" and serve with lemon wedges.

Adapted recipe from *The Candida Albicans Yeast-Free Cookbook* by Pat Connolly & Associates of the Price-Pottenger Nutrition Foundatrion (www.ppnf.org).

BEET ROOT DESSERT

YIELD: 4 SERVINGS

5 medium beets

3 medium carrots, cut into chunks

$1/4$ cup heavy whipping cream

$1/2$ teaspoon vanilla

$1/4$ teaspoon salt

1. Place the beets and carrots in a large pot and cover with water. Bring to a boil over high heat, then reduce the heat to low; cover, and simmer about 25 to 30 minutes or until the beets are tender.

2. Uncover and continue to simmer, stirring occasionally, for another 20 to 30 minutes until the liquid is reduced a bit. Remove the beets from the pot (reserve some of the cooking liquid) and set aside to cool. When the beets are cool enough to handle, peel them.

3. Transfer the beets and carrots to a food processor; add the cream, vanilla, salt, and about 2 tablespoons of the cooking liquid. Pulse until a desired texture is reached.

4. Spoon into bowls and serve.

Adapted recipe from *The Candida Albicans Yeast-Free Cookbook* by Pat Connolly & Associates of the Price-Pottenger Nutrition Foundatrion (www.ppnf.org).

Coconut Rice Pudding

YIELD: 6 TO 8 SERVINGS

2 cups cooked rice

14-ounce can coconut milk

$1/2$ teaspoon vanilla extract

$1/4$ teaspoon ground cinnamon, nutmeg, coriander, mace, or cardamom

1. Combine all the ingredients in a pot over medium-high heat. Bring to a boil, then reduce the heat to low and simmer, stirring often, for about 30 minutes or until the mixture thickens and the rice is soft and tender. If all the liquid is absorbed but the rice is still chewy, add more water, $1/4$ cup at a time, and continue to simmer until the desired texture is reached.

2. Remove from the heat and let cool a bit, then transfer to a serving bowl or individual bowls. Serve warm or refrigerate and serve chilled.

Adapted recipe from Mil Kregu; Tierra Miguel Foundation (Tierramiguelfarm.org).

Coconut Ice Cream

YIELD: 3 SERVINGS (HALF-CUP)

14-ounce can coconut milk

8 ounces heavy whipping cream

2 ounces coconut oil (optional, for added coconut taste)

1 tablespoon vanilla extract

1–2 tablespoons unsweetened coconut (optional)

1. Mix all of the ingredients together in a bowl, cover, and place in the freezer. (You can also divide the mixture in three or four small containers.) Every few hours, stir the mixture until completely frozen.

2. Before serving the ice cream, transfer it to the refrigerator for a few hours to soften it a bit.

PIE CRUST

YIELD: 9-INCH PIE CRUST

1/3 cup barley flour

1/3 cup rice flour

1/3 cup quinoa flour

1/2 cup melted butter

1. In a medium bowl, combine the flours. Add the butter and stir with a fork until it forms a crumbly, moist (not wet) dough. (If the mixture is too dry, add water a few drops at a time.) Form the dough into a ball.

2. Place the dough between two sheets of wax paper and roll it into a 10-inch circle. Transfer the circle of dough to a 9-inch pie pan and gently press it against the sides of the pan. Trim off the excess dough and crimp the edges. The crust is now ready to fill.

3. If you want to prebake the crust for a no-bake pie filling, simply prick the bottom of the dough with a fork (to keep it from bubbling up) and bake at 450°F for 10 minutes or until golden brown. Let cool before adding your favorite no-bake filling.

CONCLUSION

We all have cravings and addictions. There are life situations that upset us. However, we are responsible for what goes into our mouth as well as what comes out of our mouth, what we feel, and what we think. All of these are important to a balanced body chemistry; a body in homeostasis. Remember that if you sit down to a meal while distressed, angry, or depressed, then you are just giving yourself another kind of chocolate cake that doesn't taste as good. When you upset your body chemistry (either by negative emotions or food) you don't get the full value of the nutrients from the food that you do eat, even if it is healthy food.

CONCLUSION

A Sweet Ending Without Sugar

People starve from lack of knowledge. Actually, people do not starve—they get sick and fat from lack of knowledge. Hopefully that will not be the case for you with sugar now that you have finished this book. I'm sure many of you have identified with my story of sugar addiction, and I hope you realize that if I could break that pattern so could you.

At this point in the book, you've heard me rail against sugar and fructose. You have heard me talk about mineral relationships—especially the calcium-phosphorus ratio—that are upset by sugar, fried food, stress, and allergens. You have read my chapter on fructose being in some ways worse than table sugar, especially since fructose raises triglycerides, which has been linked to diabetes, heart disease, and cancer.

Some of you were probably not aware of the incredible amount of sugar that the average person eats in so many forms, hidden and in plain eyesight. This book should have grabbed your attention, making you realize just how much sugar you consume.

For those of you who were still not convinced at that point, you read about the disruptions to body chemistry, commonly known as diseases, that sugar causes. Showing you the consequences of overindulgence of sugar hopefully brought everyone into the fold.

All the tools for licking the sugar habit were there to read. I gave you many ideas for snacks, healthy eating habits, food plans, and recipes. I can only hope you take this new knowledge and put it to good use.

You now know that what you don't put in your mouth is as important, or more important, as what you do put in your mouth. You can sit down to a perfect meal from Food Plan III and then ruin it with a piece of chocolate cake that will cancel out the goodness of all the nutrients present in the meal. Sugar and chocolate unbalance body chemistry, making the nutrients less useful.

Sugar is the main item in our life that throws our body out of homeostasis. It is so available, so acceptable in our society, so tasty, and so addictive. I have shown you what sugar does to the body as well as many ways to remove sugar from your diet. You have all the information you need, and now it's up to you.

We all have cravings, addictions, and angry moments. However, you are responsible for what passes through your mouth in both directions. Angry words can be disruptive to body chemistry. Balance your body chemistry and keep it there.

More information about sugar can be obtained at my website, www.nancyappleton.com. I can also be reached through my website—just enter the site, click "Basic Theory" and then "Contact Us."

Health or disease, you choose.

Glossary

acetate. A salt derived from the union of acetic acid and a base or radical.

AGEs. Sugar and protein that bind nonenzymatically in the body, producing glycated protein or advanced glycation end products (AGEs). Also called glycotoxins.

albumin. Water-soluble proteins that can be coagulated by heat and are found in egg whites, blood serum, milk, and many other animal and plant tissues.

allergin. An antigenic substance capable of producing immediate type hypersensitivity or a delayed reaction (allergy).

allergy. Allergies are inappropriate or exaggerated reactions of the immune system to substances that, in the majority of people, cause no symptoms. Symptoms of the allergic diseases may be caused by a food, chemicals, dust, pollen, or other substances.

Alzheimer's disease. A brain disorder that causes problems with memory.

amino acids. The end product of protein metabolism.

anandamide. A naturally-occurring chemical compound in the brain that is released in response to pain. It also helps regulate mood, memory, and appetite.

anemia. A qualitative or quantitative deficiency of hemoglobin, a molecule found inside red blood cells.

antioxidant. An enzyme or organic substance capable of counteracting the damaging effects of oxidation.

appendicitis. Inflammation of the appendix.

atherosclerosis. Inflammation of the arteries due to the hardening of plaque on the artery walls. In some cases calcium deposits may also form. As a result of atherosclerosis, blood vessels narrow, thicken, harden, and lose elasticity; blood flow decreases; and thrombosis, heart disease, and stroke may result.

Bacteroidetes. A class of bacteria that studies have shown is less present in obese individuals. It is unknown if Bacteroidetes prevent obesity or if they simply manifest in individuals who are not obese.

biliary tract. The path by which bile is secreted by the liver on its way to the small intestine.

bulimia. An eating disorder mostly affecting young women. Bulimia is characterized by frequent excessive eating, followed by self-induced vomiting in order to avoid gaining weight.

C-peptide. An enzyme that is used as a marker on blood tests.

Candida Albicans. A form of yeast that is also a fungus. It is normally present on the skin and in mucous membranes. It can also travel through the bloodstream and affect the throat, intestines, and heart valves.

cancer. A disease in which cells in a part of the body start to grow out of control. Normally, cells grow, divide, and die in an orderly manner. Cancer cells develop due to damage to DNA. Most of the time when DNA becomes damaged, the cell can repair itself or die. In cancer cells, there is no repair, causing the normal grow, divide, die routine to become abnormal.

capillary. A minute blood vessel between the end of an artery and the beginning of a vein.

carcinogenic. Producing a malignant (cancerous) growth.

carcinoma. A form of cancer that invades surrounding tissues and organs and may spread to other places in the body.

cataract. A cloudy film covering the lens of the eye that reduces the amount of incoming light.

Crohn's disease. An inflammatory disease of the digestive system. Crohn's disease can affect any part of the digestive system, from mouth to anus.

collagen. A class of proteins in the skin, bones, cartilage, tendons, and teeth that serves as connective tissue between cells.

degenerative diseases. Diseases marked by the deterioration of a tissue, organ, or body function.

dementia. A decline in any mental function, including short- and long-term memory, logic, language, and personality.

diabetes. High blood sugar levels that result from defects in insulin secretion, action, or both.

dopamine. A neurotransmitter (messenger) found in the brain that is essential for the normal functioning of the central nervous system.

duodenal ulcer. A hole in the lining of the duodenum (the first portion of the small intestine) where it connects to the stomach.

dyspepsia. A disorder of digestive function characterized by discomfort, heartburn, or nausea.

eczema. An inflammatory skin disease characterized by tiny blisters, reddening, bumps, crusting of the skin, and thickening and scaling of the skin, causing itchiness.

emphysema. The loss of the normal elasticity of the lung that helps to hold airways open. This disease is marked by decreased ability to exhale.

endocrine system. A network of ductless glands that secrete hormones into the bloodstream.

endometrial. The layer of tissue that lines the uterus.

enzyme. A protein that acts as a catalyst to accelerate specific chemical reactions, but does not itself undergo any change during the reaction. Digestive enzymes break down complex carbohydrates into simple sugars, fats or lipids into fatty acids, and protein into amino acids.

estradiol. One of the forms of naturally-occurring estrogen that is produced by the body.

etiology. The study of causation.

fermentation. The conversion of sugar to carbon dioxide or alcohol by yeast.

Firmicutes. A class of bacteria that studies have associated with obesity, since these bacteria generally have a larger presence in obese individuals.

flavanols. An antioxidant found in cocoa beans that can increase blood flow to the brain.

free radical. An atom or group of atoms that has at least one unpaired electron and is therefore unstable and highly reactive. In animal tissues, free radicals can damage cells and are believed to accelerate the progression of cancer, cardiovascular disease, and age-related diseases.

fructose. A form of sugar that is found in many foods. It is also derived from the digestion of granulated table sugar (sucrose) and corn sweetener, which is made up of glucose and fructose.

functional bowel disease. A gastrointestinal disorder specific to the mid or lower gastrointestinal tract.

gallstone. A solid material formed in the gallbladder or bile duct. A gallstone is usually composed of cholesterol, calcium salts, and bile pigments. There are many different treatment options for gallstones, including surgery, medicine, or a self-administered "gallbladder flush."

gastric cancer. Cancer of or relating to the stomach.

gastric ulcers. Also called a stomach ulcer. A gastric ulcer is an eroded area in the lining of the stomach.

gestation duration. The length of time of a pregnancy.

ghrelin. A hormone produced in the stomach and pancreas that stimulates appetite.

glucose. A simple sugar (monosaccharide), also called dextrose or grape sugar, which is found in fruits, vegetables, tree sap, sucrose, honey, corn syrup, and molasses. Glucose provides most of the energy for the cells of the body.

glycation. A condition in which sugar and protein are bound nonenzymatically in the body. This can disrupt the body chemistry

glycemic index. A numerical system measuring how quickly a food triggers a rise in blood glucose.

glycemic load. A method of assessing the impact carbohydrate consumption will have on blood glucose. The glycemic load, unlike the glycemic index, takes serving size into account when determining a food's effect on blood glucose.

glycoprotein. Any part of a group of complex proteins that contain a carbohydrate combined with a protein.

gout. A disease involving inflammation of the joints, especially in the hands and feet. Gout is also associated with an excess of uric acid in the blood.

HDL (high density lipoprotein). A protein in blood plasma that carries cholesterol and other fats from the blood to the tissues.

heart arrhythmia. A heart rhythm problem. Heart arrhythmias are common and usually harmless, but some can lead to life-threatening conditions.

heart disease. Conditions affecting the heart, such as coronary heart disease, heart attack, and heart failure. It is the leading cause of death for men and women in the United States.

hemorrhoid. An enlarged vein (usually due to an increase in venous pressure) occurring inside the anal sphincter (internal hemorrhoid) or outside the anal sphincter (external hemorrhoid).

high-fructose corn syrup. A sweetener made up of any group of corn syrups that has undergone processing to increase its fructose content. This sweetener is used in almost all processed foods and beverages, including soft drinks, ketchup, yogurt, cookies, and salad dressing.

hives. Red, itchy bumps on the skin, usually caused by an allergic reaction.

homeostasis. A balance of all body functions and systems. When homeostasis is impaired, the stage is set for disease.

homocysteine. A naturally-occurring amino acid found in blood plasma. High levels of homocysteine in the blood are believed to increase the chance of heart disease, stroke, Alzheimer's disease, and osteoporosis.

hormone. A chemical released by a cell that affects the function of organs or tissues in the body.

hyperglycemia. High blood sugar.

hypertension. High blood pressure.

hypoglycemia. Low blood sugar.

immune system. A collection of cells and proteins that works to protect the body from potentially harmful, infectious microorganisms (microscopic life-forms), such as bacteria, viruses, and fungi. The immune system plays a role in the control of cancer and other diseases, but also is the culprit in the phenomena of allergies, hypersensitivity, and the rejection of transplanted organs, tissues, and medical implants.

infectious diseases. Diseases caused by the invasion of bacteria, virus, or other agent.

inflammation. Redness, swelling, pain, and disturbed function in an area of the body.

insulin. A hormone made by the pancreas that controls the level of the sugar (glucose) in the blood. Insulin permits cells to use glucose for energy. Cells cannot utilize glucose without insulin.

insulin resistance. A condition in which normal amounts of insulin are not adequate to produce a normal insulin response.

irritable bowel syndrome (IBS). A functional bowel disorder characterized by mild to severe abdominal pain, bloating, discomfort, and abnormal bowel movements. Some cases involve diarrhea, while others involve constipation or a combination of the two. Sometimes the symptoms can be relieved by bowel movements.

ketogenic diet. A diet of mostly fat and protein with some vegetables. Absolutely no sugar is allowed for people on this diet.

lactic acid. A chemical compound that is a byproduct of glucose. Lactic acid accumulates in the muscles after vigorous exercise prevents adequate oxygen intake. Lactic acid makes the muscles hurt and causes fatigue.

lactose. The sugar found in milk. The body uses the enzyme lactase to break down lactose into galactose and glucose.

laryngeal cancer. Cancer of the larynx, also known as the voicebox.

larynx. Known as the voicebox, it is an organ involved in the protection of the trachea and sound production.

LDL (low density lipoproteins). The portion of blood containing large amounts of cholesterol and triglycerides. Elevated LDLs are implicated in heart disease.

leptin. A hormone that plays a key role in energy intake and expenditure.

lipid. An organic substance; a fat.

lipoprotein. A biochemical structure made up of a lipid and a protein. Lipoproteins transport lipids throughout the body.

macular degeneration. A loss of vision in the center of the eye that can lead to blindness.

Maillard reaction. A reaction between an amino acid and a sugar, usually requiring heat. The Maillard reaction is a form of nonenzymatic food browning.

maltodextrin. A sweet, easily digested carbohydrate often made from cornstarch that is digested and absorbed rapidly, and therefore has a high glycemic index. It is used as a food additive.

metabolic syndrome. A disease classified by a group of metabolic risk factors, including obesity, high blood pressure, insulin resistance, and others.

metabolism. Chemical processes occurring within a living organism or cell that are necessary to maintain life.

minerals. Elements taken from food that are crucial to the functioning of the human body.

multiple sclerosis (MS). A disease that attacks the central nervous system, which can have minor symptoms, such as numbness of the limbs, or severe symptoms, such as paralysis or loss of vision. The progress, severity, and specific symptoms of the disease are unpredictable.

myopia. An eye defect where people can see nearby objects, but distant objects appear blurry. Also called nearsightedness.

neural tube defects. A major birth defect caused by abnormal development of the neural tube, which is the structure in an embryo from which the brain and spinal cord form.

neuron. A nerve encompassing the cell and the long fiber originating from the cell.

neurotransmitter. Chemical messenger that works throughout the body.

norepinephrine. Both a hormone and a neurotransmitter. As a hormone, it is secreted by the adrenal gland and works alongside epinephrine and adrenaline to give the body energy in times of stress. This is known as the "fight or flight" response. As a neurotransmitter, it passes nerve impulses from one neuron to the next.

osteoporosis. The loss of bone or skeletal tissue producing brittleness or softness of bone.

oxidative stress. Occurs when the available supply of the body's antioxidants is insufficient to handle and neutralize free radicals of different types. The result is massive cell damage that can result in cellular mutations, tissue breakdown, and immune compromise.

pathological changes. Disease-causing changes.

periodontal disease. Disease of the tissues surrounding the teeth.

pH. A scale denoting the acidity or alkalinity of a solution.

phenylethylamine. A chemical that raises blood pressure and blood glucose levels. It is referred to as the "love drug," because it mimics the brain chemistry of a person in love.

phosphatase. Any of various enzymes found in body tissues and fluids that hydrolyze phosphoric acid esters of organic compounds, liberating phosphate ions.

pilocarpine. A drug that mimics the effects of a chemical that serves as a messenger between nerve cells and the organs they control.

plasma. The clear, yellowish, liquid portion of blood.

platelet adhesiveness. A term used to describe the situation in which platelets adhere to something other than platelets.

polio. A viral disease involving inflammation of the nerve cells in the brain and spinal cord.

polypeptides. Intermediate state of protein breakdown. Polypeptides can do harm if they enter the bloodstream before they are broken down into amino acids.

positron emission tomography (PET) scans. A type of imaging that allows doctors to see how organs and tissues inside the body are actually functioning.

postoperative stress. Discomfort and/or pain during the recovery period after an operation.

pre-diabetes. A condition where blood glucose is higher than normal, but not high enough to be classified as type-2 diabetes.

premature aging. Premature aging of the brain, circulation system, heart, joints, digestive tract, and immune system can begin at any time in life. Various factors cause the body to deteriorate, including injuries that do not heal completely, allergies, toxic chemicals, poor nutrition, excessive radiation sunlight, overwhelming stress, and inactivity.

proteolytic enzymes. Enzymes from the pancreas that aid in the digestion of proteins into amino acids.

psoriasis. A skin condition consisting of gray or silvery flaky patches on the skin, which is red and inflamed.

purine. A white, crystalline compound, from which a number of compounds are derived, including uric acid and caffeine.

reward system. A psychological reward is a process that reinforces behavior—something that, when offered, causes a behavior to increase in intensity.

rheumatoid arthritis. An inflammatory form of arthritis that causes joint pain and soreness.

schizophrenia. A chronic, severe brain disorder. Sufferers sometimes hear voices others do not hear, believe others are broadcasting their thoughts, or become convinced that people are trying to harm or sabotage them. This can make sufferers withdrawn or fearful. Symptoms can include hallucinations, delusions, and social withdrawal.

seizure. A sudden attack, convulsion, or spasm; as seen in people who suffer from epilepsy.

serotonin. A neurotransmitter that plays a role in sleep, depression, and memory.

serum. A clear, yellowish substance obtained from separating the liquid part of blood from the solid part of blood when blood clots.

sucrose. Sugar derived from sugarcane or beet; also known as table sugar.

sugar alcohols. Carbohydrates mostly manufactured from sugars and starches.

tissue elasticity. The tension (pressure) required to produce elongation (stretching).

total parenteral nutrition. Intravenous feeding that provides a patient with all of the fluids and essential nutrients he or she needs when unable to feed him or herself by mouth.

toxemia. A serious medical condition that usually affects the women who contract it after twenty weeks of pregnancy. Also known as preeclampsia or pregnancy-induced hypertension, toxemia is characterized by sudden elevated blood pressure and the presence of excess protein in the urine.

triglycerides. This class of fats makes up most animal and vegetable fats and appears in the blood bound to a protein, forming high and low-density lipoproteins.

Ulcerative colitis. A disease that causes inflammation and sores, called ulcers, in the lining of the rectum and colon.

ulcers. Sores on the lining of your digestive tract.

uremia. Buildup of waste products in the blood due to the kidney's inability to excrete them.

uric acid. A product of purines, which are found in many foods. Uric acid is the final oxidation (breakdown) product of purine metabolism, and it is excreted in urine.

urinary electrolyte composition. A urine test that measures chemicals (electrolytes) in urine. It usually measures the levels of calcium, chloride, potassium, or sodium.

varicose veins. Gnarled, enlarged veins.

VLDL (very low-density lipoprotein). VLDL cholesterol is one of the three major types of lipoproteins. The other two are high-density lipoprotein (HDL) cholesterol and low-density lipoprotein (LDL) cholesterol. Each type contains a mixture of cholesterol, protein, and triglyceride, but in varying amounts.

Resources

Associations and Organizations

American Association of Pediatrics
141 Northwest Point Boulevard
Elk Grove Village, IL 60007
Phone: (847) 434-4000
Website: (www.aap.org/)
The American Association of Pediatrics (AAP) is committed to the attainment of optimal physical, mental, and social health and well-being for all infants, children, adolescents, and young adults.

American Diabetes Association
ATTN: National Call Center
1701 North Beauregard Street
Alexandria, VA 22311
Phone: 1-800-DIABETES (342-2383)
Website: (www.diabetes.org/home.jsp)
The American Diabetes Association is leading the fight against the deadly consequences of diabetes and fighting for those affected by diabetes. The Association funds research to prevent, cure, and manage diabetes; delivers services to hundreds of communities; provides objective and credible information; and gives voice to those denied their rights because of diabetes.

American Society for Nutrition
American Journal of Clinical Nutrition
9650 Rockville Pike
Bethesda, MD 20814
Phone: (301) 634-7050
Website: (www.nutrition.org/)
Website for *American Journal of Clinical Nutrition:* (www.ajcn.org/)
The American Society for Nutrition (ASN) is a non-profit organization dedicated to bringing together the world's top researchers, clinical nutritionists, and industry to advance our knowledge and application of nutrition for the sake of humans and animals. Their focus ranges from the most critical details of research and application to the broadest applications in society, in the United States and around the world.

Beech-Nut
Phone: 1-800-BEECH-NUT (233-2468)
Website: (www.beechnut.comindex.asp)
Beech-Nut has been making natural, great-tasting baby food for over seventy-five years. They have their own test kitchen where they taste the food they produce to make sure it's healthy and delicious. They use high-quality, all-natural ingredients plus vitamins and minerals to make their food so you know that when you choose Beech-Nut, you're making a better choice.

Center for Science in the Public Interest
1875 Connecticut Avenue, NW, Suite 300
Washington, DC 20009
Phone: (202) 332-9110
Website: (www.cspinet.org/index.html)
Since 1971, the Center for Science in the Public Interest (CSPI) has been a strong advocate for nutrition and health, food safety, alcohol policy, and sound science. CSPI carved out a niche as the organized voice of the American public on nutrition, food safety, health, and other issues during a boom of consumer and environmental protection awareness in the early 1970s. CSPI has long sought to educate the public, advocate government policies that are consistent with scientific evidence on health and environmental issues, and counter industry's powerful influence on public opinion and public policies.

The Epilepsy Foundation
8301 Professional Place
Landover, MD 20785
Phone: (800) 332-1000
Website: (www.epilepsyfoundation.org/)
The Epilepsy Foundation of America is the national voluntary agency solely dedicated to the welfare of the more than 3 million people with epilepsy in the United States and their families. The organization works to ensure that people with seizures are able to participate in all life experiences; to improve how people with epilepsy are perceived, accepted and valued in society; and to promote research for a cure.

Food Addicts Anonymous
4623 Forest Hill Boulevard, Suite 109-4
West Palm Beach, FL 33415
Phone: (561) 967-3871
Website: (www.foodaddictsanonymous.org/)
Food Addicts Anonymous (FAA) is a fellowship of men and women who are willing to recover from the disease of food addiction. Sharing their experience, strength, and hope with others allows addicts to recover from this disease, one day at a time.

Food Addicts in Recovery Anonymous
40 W. Cummings Park #1700
Woburn, MA 01801
Phone: (781) 932-6300
Website: (http://foodaddicts.org/index.html)
Food Addicts in Recovery Anonymous (FA) is an international fellowship of men and women who have experienced difficulties in life as a result of the way they eat. Members join FA either because they could not control their eating or because they were obsessed with food. FA's program of recovery is based on the Twelve Steps and Twelve Traditions of Alcoholics Anonymous. They make use of AA principles to gain freedom from addictive eating. There are no dues, fees, or weigh-ins at FA meetings. Membership is open to anyone who wants help with food.

Harvard Health Publications
Phone: (877) 649-9457
Website: (https://www.health.harvard.edu/)
Website for glycemic index information: (https://www.health.harvard.edu/newsweek/Glycemic_index_and_glycemic_load_for_100_foods.htm)
Harvard Health Publications is a division of the Harvard Medical School. The goal of the publications is to bring to the public, around the world, the most current, practical, authoritative health information, drawing on the expertise of the 8,000 faculty physicians at the Harvard Medical School and its world-famous affiliated hospitals.

Healthy Kids, Smart Kids
Phone: (770) 617-6587
Website: (www.healthykidssmartkids.comindex.htm)
Healthy Kids, Smart Kids is a school and family healthy lifestyle plan that's making a real difference. Over 9 million U.S. children are overweight or obese. Studies show nutrition and exercise can help improve health and grades. Their goal is to build a sustainable, measurable wellness program for schools and families.

The Hypoglycemia Support Foundation, Inc.
P.O. Box 451778
Sunrise, FL 33345
Website: (www.hypoglycemia.org/default.asp)
The Hypoglycemia Support Foundation, Inc., works to inform, support, and encourage hypoglycemics and the public about this too often misunderstood and misdiagnosed disease. The organization shows how poor nutritional habits and severe nutritional deficiencies affect one's emotional and physical health.

Johns Hopkins Bloomberg School of Public Health
615 N. Wolfe Street
Baltimore, MD 21205
Phone: (410) 955-3847
Website: (www.jhsph.edu/)
Website for obesity information: (www.jhsph.edu/publichealthnews/press_releases/2007/wang_adult_obesity.html)
The Johns Hopkins Bloomberg School of Public Health is dedicated

to the education of a diverse group of research scientists and public health professionals, a process inseparably linked to the discovery and application of new knowledge, and through these activities, to the improvement of health and prevention of disease and disability around the world.

National Heart, Lung, and Blood Institute

Building 31, Room 5A52
31 Center Drive MSC 2486
Bethesda, MD 20892
Phone: (301) 592-8573
Website: (www.nhlbi.nih.gov/index.htm)
Website for BMI calculation information: (www.nhlbisupport.combmi/)
The National Heart, Lung, and Blood Institute (NHLBI) provides leadership for a national program in diseases of the heart, blood vessels, lung, and blood; blood resources; and sleep disorders. Since October 1997, the NHLBI has also had administrative responsibility for the NIH Woman's Health Initiative.

National Institute of Mental Health

Science Writing, Press, and Dissemination Branch
6001 Executive Boulevard, Room 8184, MSC 9663
Bethesda, MD 20892
Phone: (866) 615-6464
Website: (www.nimh.nih.gov/index.shtml)
The National Institute of Mental Health (NIMH) envisions a world in which mental illnesses are prevented and cured. The mission of NIMH is to transform the understanding and treatment of mental illnesses through basic and clinical research, paving the way for prevention, recovery, and cure.

Robert Wood Johnson Foundation

P.O. Box 2316
Route 1 and College Road East
Princeton, NJ 08543
Phone: (877) 843-RWJF (7953)
Website: (http://www.rwjf.org)
The mission of the Robert Wood Johnson Foundation (RWJF) is to improve the health and heathcare of all Americans. Their goal is to help Americans lead healthier lives and get the care they need.

U.S. Department of Agriculture
Agricultural Research Service
Jamie L. Whitten Building
1400 Independence Avenue, SW
Washington, DC 20250
Phone: (301) 504-6078
Website: (www.ars.usda.gov/main/main.htm)
Website for information pertaining to added sugars:
  (www.ars.usda.gov/Services/docs.htm?docid=12107)
The Agricultural Research Service (ARS) is the U.S. Department of Agriculture's chief scientific research agency. Its job is finding solutions to agricultural problems that affect Americans every day, from field to table.

Websites

The following websites all contain information about the glycemic index and glycemic load.

Calorie Count (http://caloriecount.about.com)
Calorie Count was created to provide you with all the guidance and support you need for a healthy lifestyle — one that you'll enjoy leading every day.

The Calorie Counter (www.thecaloriecounter.com)
The calorie counter provides a way to count your daily caloric intake with its easy-to-use calorie counter. Calorie counting is an easy way for you to manage your weight. If you have a daily caloric requirement that you want to meet, or you need to monitor your caloric intake, its calorie counting technique is for you.

Home of the Glycemic Index (www.glycemicindex.com)
Home of the Glycemic Index is the official website for the glycemic index and international GI database which is based in the Human Nutrition Unit, School of Molecular and Microbial Biosciences, University of Sydney. The website is updated and maintained by the University's GI Group, which includes research scientists and dietitians working in the area of glycemic index, health, and nutrition, including research into diet and weight loss, diabetes, cardiovascular disease, and PCOS.

Nutrition Data (www.nutritiondata.com)

Since its launch in 2003, Nutrition Data has grown into one of the most authoritative and useful sources of nutritional analysis on the Web. In July 2006, Nutrition Data was acquired by CondéNet, a digital publisher under the Condé Nast Publications umbrella dedicated to editorial excellence. Nutrition Data's continuing goal is to provide the most accurate and comprehensive nutrition analysis available, and to make it accessible and understandable to all.

Recommended Reading

These books are filled with important information. They will add to the information on sugar and they will be useful to the people who need further help after removing sugar from their diet. All books are available through Amazon, www.amazon.com.

Brain Allergies, by Dr. William Philpott

The Do's and Don'ts of Hypoglycemia: An Everyday Guide to Low Blood Sugar, by Roberta Ruggerio

The Wisdom of the Body, by Walter B. Cannon, MD, PhD

Notes

Chapter 1

1. Avena, N.N. et al. "Evidence for addiction: behavioral and neurochemical effects of intermittent, excessive sugar intake." *Neurosci Biobehav Rev.* 2008; 32(1): 20–39.

2. Lenoir, M. et al. "Intense Sweetness Surpasses Cocaine Reward." *PLoS One.* Aug 1, 2007; 2(1): e698.

3. U.S. Department of Agriculture. "Food Availability: Custom Queries." www.ers.usda.gov/Data/FoodConsumption/FoodAvailQueriable.aspx.

Chapter 2

Please note that citations for this chapter correspond to their respective numbers on the list, and that some of the listed reasons have more than one reference.

1. Sanchez, A., et al. "Role of Sugars in Human Neutrophilic Phagocytosis." *Am J Clin Nutr.* Nov 1973; 261: 1180–1184.

2. Bernstein, J., et al. "Depression of Lymphocyte Transformation Following Oral Glucose Ingestion." *Am J Clin Nutr.* 1997; 30: 613.

3. Schauss, A. *Diet, Crime and Delinquency.* (Berkley, CA: Parker House, 1981).

4. Bayol, S.A. "Evidence that a Maternal 'Junk Food' Diet during Pregnancy and Lactation Can Reduce Muscle Force in Offspring." *Eur J Nutr.* Dec 19, 2008.

5. Rajeshwari, R., et al."Secular Trends in Children's Sweetened-beverage Consumption (1973 to 1994): The Bogalusa Heart Study." *J Am Diet Assoc.* Feb 2005; 105(2): 208–214.

6. Behall, K. "Influence of Estrogen Content of Oral Contraceptives and Consumption of Sucrose on Blood Parameters." *Disease Abstracts International.* 1982; 431–437. POPLINE Document Number: 013114.

7. Mohanty, P., et al. "Glucose Challenge Stimulates Reactive Oxygen Species (ROS) Generation by Leucocytes." *J Clin Endocrin Metab.* Aug 2000; 85(8): 2970–2973.

    Couzy, F., et al."Nutritional Implications of the Interaction Minerals." *Progressive Food & Nutrition Science.* 1933; 17: 65–87.

8. Goldman, J., et al. "Behavioral Effects of Sucrose on Preschool Children." *J Abnorm Child Psy.* 1986; 14(4): 565–577.

9. Scanto, S. and Yudkin, J. "The Effect of Dietary Sucrose on Blood Lipids, Serum Insulin, Platelet Adhesiveness and Body Weight in Human Volunteers." *Postgrad Med J.* 1969; 45: 602–607.

10. Ringsdorf, W., Cheraskin, E., and Ramsay, R. "Sucrose, Neutrophilic Phagocytosis and Resistance to Disease." *Dental Survey.* 1976; 52(12): 46–48.

11. Cerami, A., et al. "Glucose and Aging." *Scientific American.* May 1987: 90.

   Lee, A. T. and Cerami, A. "The Role of Glycation in Aging." *Annals N Y Acad Sci.* 663: 63–67.

12. Albrink, M. and Ullrich, I.H. "Interaction of Dietary Sucrose and Fiber on Serum Lipids in Healthy Young Men Fed High Carbohydrate Diets." *Clin Nutr.* 1986; 43: 419–428.

   Pamplona, R., et al. "Mechanisms of Glycation in Atherogenesis." *Medical Hypotheses.* Mar 1993; 40(3): 174–81.

13. Kozlovsky, A., et al. "Effects of Diets High in Simple Sugars on Urinary Chromium Losses." *Metabolism.* Jun 1986; 35: 515–518.

14. Takahashi, E. Tohoku, University School of Medicine. *Wholistic Health Digest.* Oct 1982: 41.

15. Kelsay, J., et al. "Diets High in Glucose or Sucrose and Young Women." *Am J Clin Nutr.* 1974; 27: 926–936.

   Thomas, B. J., et al. "Relation of Habitual Diet to Fasting Plasma Insulin Concentration and the Insulin Response to Oral Glucose." *Hum Nutr Clin Nutr.* 1983; 36C(1): 49–51.

16. Fields, M., et al. "Effect of Copper Deficiency on Metabolism and Mortality in Rats Fed Sucrose or Starch Diets." *Am J Clin Nutr.* 1983; 113: 1335–1345.

17. Lemann, J. "Evidence that Glucose Ingestion Inhibits Net Renal Tubular Reabsorption of Calcium and Magnesium." *Am J Clin Nutr.* 1976; 70: 236–245.

18. Chiu, C. "Association between Dietary Glycemic Index and Age-related Macular Degeneration in Nondiabetic Participants in the Age-Related Eye Disease Study." *Am J Clin Nutr.* Jul 2007; 86: 180–188.

19. "Sugar, White Flour Withdrawal Produces Chemical Response." *The Addiction Letter.* Jul 1992: 4.

20. Dufty, William. *Sugar Blues.* (New York: Warner Books, 1975).

21. Ibid.

22. Jones, T.W., et al. "Enhanced Adrenomedullary Response and Increased Susceptibility to Neuroglygopenia: Mechanisms Underlying the Adverse Effect of Sugar Ingestion in Children." *J Ped.* Feb 1995; 126: 171–177.

23. Ibid.

24. Lee, A. T. and Cerami, A. "The Role of Glycation in Aging." *Annals N Y Acad Sci.* 1992; 663: 63–70.

25. Abrahamson, E. and Peget, A. *Body, Mind and Sugar.* (New York: Avon, 1977).

26. Glinsmann, W., et al. "Evaluation of Health Aspects of Sugar Contained in Carbohydrate Sweeteners." *F.D.A. Report of Sugars Task Force.* 1986: 39.

Makinen, K.K., et al. "A Descriptive Report of the Effects of a 16-month Xylitol Chewing-Gum Programme Subsequent to a 40–Month Sucrose Gum Programme." *Caries Res.* 1998; 32(2): 107–12.

Riva Touger-Decker and Cor van Loveren, "Sugars and Dental Caries." *Am J Clin Nutr.* Oct 2003; 78: 881–892.

27. Keen, H., et al. "Nutrient Intake, Adiposity, and Diabetes." *Brit Med J.* 1989; 1: 655–658.

28. Tragnone, A., et al. "Dietary Habits as Risk Factors for Inflammatory Bowel Disease." *Eur J Gastroenterol Hepatol.* Jan 1995; 7(1): 47–51.

29. Yudkin, J. *Sweet and Dangerous.* (New York: Bantam Books: 1974) 129.

30. Darlington, L., and Ramsey, et al. "Placebo-Controlled, Blind Study of Dietary Manipulation Therapy in Rheumatoid Arthritis," *Lancet.* Feb 1986; 8475(1): 236–238.

31. Schauss, A. *Diet, Crime and Delinquency.* (Berkley, CA: Parker House, 1981).

32. Crook, W. J. *The Yeast Connection.* (TN: Professional Books, 1984).

33. Heaton, K. "The Sweet Road to Gallstones." *Brit Med J.* Apr 14, 1984; 288: 1103–1104.

Misciagna, G., et al."Insulin and Gallstones." *Am J Clin Nutr.* 1999; 69: 120–126.

34. Yudkin, J. "Sugar Consumption and Myocardial Infarction." *Lancet.* Feb 6, 1971; 1(7693): 296–297.

Chess, D.J., et al. "Deleterious Effects of Sugar and Protective Effects of Starch on Cardiac Remodeling, Contractile Dysfunction, and Mortality in Response to Pressure Overload." *Am J Physiol Heart Circ Physiol.* Sep 2007; 293(3): H1853–H1860.

35. Cleave, T. *The Saccharine Disease.* (New Canaan, CT: Keats Publishing, 1974).

36. Ibid.

37. Cleave, T. and Campbell, G. *Diabetes, Coronary Thrombosis and the Saccharine Disease.* (Bristol, England: John Wright and Sons, 1960).

38. Glinsmann, W., et al. "Evaluation of Health Aspects of Sugar Contained in Carbohydrate Sweeteners." *F.D.A. Report of Sugars Task Force.* 1986; 39: 36–38.

39. Tjäderhane, L. and Larmas, M. "A High Sucrose Diet Decreases the Mechanical Strength of Bones in Growing Rats." *J Nutr.* 1998; 128: 1807–1810.

40. Wilson, R.F. and Ashley, F.P. "The Effects of Experimental Variations in Dietary

Sugar Intake and Oral Hygiene on the Biochemical Composition and pH of Free Smooth-surface and Approximal Plaque." *J Dent Res.* Jun 1988; 67(6): 949–953.

41. Beck-Nielsen, H., et al. "Effects of Diet on the Cellular Insulin Binding and the Insulin Sensitivity in Young Healthy Subjects." *Diabetes.* 1978; 15: 289–296.

42. Mohanty, P., et al. "Glucose Challenge Stimulates Reactive Oxygen Species (ROS) Generation by Leucocytes." *J Clin Endocrin Metab.* Aug 2000; 85(8): 2970–2973.

43. Gardner, L. and Reiser, S. "Effects of Dietary Carbohydrate on Fasting Levels of Human Growth Hormone and Cortisol." *Proc Soc Exp Biol Med.* 1982; 169: 36–40.

44. Ma, Y., et al. "Association Between Carbohydrate Intake and Serum Lipids." *J Am Coll Nutr.* Apr 2006; 25(2): 155–163.

45. Furth, A. and Harding, J. "Why Sugar Is Bad For You." *New Scientist.* Sep 23, 1989; 44.

46. Lee, A.T. and Cerami, A. "Role of Glycation in Aging." *Annals N Y Acad Sci.* Nov 21, 1992; 663: 63–70.

47. Appleton, N. *Lick the Sugar Habit.* (New York: Avery Penguin Putnam, 1988).

48. Henriksen, H. B. and Kolset, S.O. *Tidsskr Nor Laegeforen.* Sep 6, 2007; 127(17): 2259–62.

49. Cleave, T. *The Saccharine Disease.* (New Canaan, CT: Keats Publishing, 1974).

50. Ibid., at 132.

51. Vaccaro, O., et al. "Relationship of Postload Plasma Glucose to Mortality with 19 Year Follow-up." *Diabetes Care.* Oct 15,1992; 10: 328–334.

   Tominaga, M., et al, "Impaired Glucose Tolerance Is a Risk Factor for Cardiovascular Disease, but Not Fasting Glucose." *Diabetes Care.* 1999; 2(6): 920–924.

52. Lee, A. T. and Cerami, A. "Modifications of Proteins and Nucleic Acids by Reducing Sugars: Possible Role in Aging." *Handbook of the Biology of Aging.* (New York: Academic Press, 1990).

53. Monnier, V. M. "Nonenzymatic Glycosylation, the Maillard Reaction and the Aging Process." *J Ger.* 1990; 45(4): 105–110.

54. Dyer, D. G., et al. "Accumulation of Maillard Reaction Products in Skin Collagen in Diabetes and Aging." *J Clin Invest.* 1993; 93(6): 421–422.

55. Veromann, S., et al. "Dietary Sugar and Salt Represent Real Risk Factors for Cataract Development." *Ophthalmologica.* Jul-Aug 2003; 217(4): 302–307.

56. Monnier, V. M. "Nonenzymatic Glycosylation, the Maillard Reaction and the Aging Process." *J Ger.* 1990; 45(4): 105–110.

57. Schmidt, A.M., et al. "Activation of Receptor for Advanced Glycation End Products: a Mechanism for Chronic Vascular Dysfunction in Diabetic Vasculopathy and Atherosclerosis." *Circ Res.* Mar 1999; 1984(5): 489–97.

58. Lewis, G. F. and Steiner, G. "Acute Effects of Insulin in the Control of VLDL Production in Humans. Implications for The Insulin-resistant State." *Diabetes Care.* Apr 1996; 19(4): 390–393.

R. Pamplona, M.J., et al. "Mechanisms of Glycation in Atherogenesis." *Medical Hypotheses.* 1990; 40: 174–181.

59. Ceriello, A. "Oxidative Stress and Glycemic Regulation." *Metabolism.* Feb 2000; 49(2 Suppl 1): 27–29.

60. Appleton, Nancy. *Lick the Sugar Habit.* (New York: Avery Penguin Putnam, 1988).

61. Hellenbrand, W., et al. "Diet and Parkinson's Disease. A Possible Role for the Past Intake of Specific Nutrients. Results from a Self-administered Food-frequency Questionnaire in a Case-control Study." *Neurology.* Sep 1996; 47: 644–650.

Cerami, A., et al. "Glucose and Aging." *Sci Am.* May 1987: 90.

62. Goulart, F. S. "Are You Sugar Smart?" *American Fitness.* Mar-Apr 1991: 34–38.

63. Scribner, K.B., et al. "Hepatic Steatosis and Increased Adiposity in Mice Consuming Rapidly vs. Slowly Absorbed Carbohydrate." *Obesity.* 2007; 15: 2190–2199.

64. Yudkin, J., Kang, S., and Bruckdorfer, K. "Effects of High Dietary Sugar." *Brit Med J.* Nov 22, 1980; 1396.

65. Goulart, F. S. "Are You Sugar Smart?" *American Fitness.* Mar-Apr 1991: 34–38

66. Ibid.

67. Ibid.

68. Ibid.

69. Ibid.

70. Nash, J. "Health Contenders." *Essence.* Jan 1992; 23: 79–81.

71. Grand, E. "Food Allergies and Migraine." *Lancet.* 1979; 1: 955–959.

72. Michaud, D. "Dietary Sugar, Glycemic Load, and Pancreatic Cancer Risk in a Prospective Study." *J Natl Cancer Inst.* Sep 4, 2002; 94(17): 1293–300.

73. Schauss, A. *Diet, Crime and Delinquency.* (Berkley, CA: Parker House, 1981).

74. Peet, M. "International Variations in the Outcome of Schizophrenia and the Prevalence of Depression in Relation to National Dietary Practices: An Ecological Analysis." *Brit J Psy.* 2004; 184: 404–408.

75. Cornee, J., et al. "A Case-control Study of Gastric Cancer and Nutritional Factors in Marseille, France." *Eur J Epid.* 1995; 11: 55–65.

76. Yudkin, J. *Sweet and Dangerous.* (New York: Bantam Books, 1974).

77. Ibid., at 44.

78. Reiser, S., et al. "Effects of Sugars on Indices on Glucose Tolerance in Humans." *Am J Clin Nutr.* 1986: 43; 151–159.

79. Ibid.

Molteni, R., et al. "A High-fat, Refined Sugar Diet Reduces Hippocampal Brain-derived Neurotrophic Factor, Neuronal Plasticity, and Learning." *NeuroScience.* 2002; 112(4): 803–814.

80. Monnier, V., "Nonenzymatic Glycosylation, the Maillard Reaction and the Aging Process." *J Ger.* 1990; 45: 105–111.

81. Frey, J. "Is There Sugar in the Alzheimer's Disease?" *Annales De Biologie Clinique.* 2001; 59(3): 253–257.

82. Yudkin, J. "Metabolic Changes Induced by Sugar in Relation to Coronary Heart Disease and Diabetes." *Nutr Health.* 1987; 5(1–2): 5–8.

83. Ibid.

84. Blacklock, N.J., "Sucrose and Idiopathic Renal Stone." *Nutr Health.* 1987; 5(1–2):9–12. Curhan, G., et al. "Beverage Use and Risk for Kidney Stones in Women." *Ann Inter Med.* 1998; 28: 534–340.

85. Ceriello, A. "Oxidative Stress and Glycemic Regulation." *Metabolism.* Feb 2000; 49(2 Suppl 1): 27–29.

86. Moerman, C. J., et al. "Dietary Sugar Intake in the Etiology of Biliary Tract Cancer." *Inter J Epid.* Apr 1993; 2(2): 207–214.

87. Lenders, C. M. "Gestational Age and Infant Size at Birth Are Associated with Dietary Intake among Pregnant Adolescents." *J Nutr.* Jun 1997; 1113–1117.

88. Ibid.

89. Yudkin, J. and Eisa, O. "Dietary Sucrose and Oestradiol Concentration in Young Men." *Ann Nutr Metab.* 1988; 32(2): 53–55.

90. Bostick, R.M., et al. "Sugar, Meat, and Fat Intake and Non-dietary Risk Factors for Colon Cancer Incidence in Iowa Women." *Cancer Causes & Control.* 1994; 5: 38–53.

Kruis, W., et al. "Effects of Diets Low and High in Refined Sugars on Gut Transit, Bile Acid Metabolism and Bacterial Fermentation." *Gut.* 1991; 32: 367–370.

Ludwig, D. S., et al. "High Glycemic Index Foods, Overeating, And Obesity." *Pediatrics.* Mar 1999; 103(3): 26–32.

91. Yudkin, J. and Eisa, O. "Dietary Sucrose and Oestradiol Concentration in Young Men." *Ann Nutr Metab.* 1988; 32(2): 53–55.

92. Lee, A.T. and Cerami, A. "The Role of Glycation in Aging." *Annals N Y Acad Sci.* 1992; 663: 63–70.

93. Moerman, C., et al."Dietary Sugar Intake in the Etiology of Gallbladder Tract Cancer." *Inter J Epid.* Apr 1993; 22(2): 207–214.

94. Avena, N.M. "Evidence for Sugar Addiction: Behavioral and Nuerochemical Effects of Intermittent, Excessive Sugar Intake." *Neurosci Biobehav Rev.* 2008; 32(1): 20–39.

Colantuoni, C., et al. "Evidence That Intermittent, Excessive Sugar Intake Cause Endogenous Opioid Dependence." *Obesity.* Jun 2002; 10(6): 478–488.

95. Ibid.

96. *The Edell Health Letter.* Sep 1991; 7: 1.

97. Christensen, L., et al. "Impact of A Dietary Change on Emotional Distress." *J Abnorm Psy.* 1985; 94(4): 565–79.

98. Ludwig, D.S., et al. "High Glycemic Index Foods, Overeating and Obesity." *Pediatrics.* Mar 1999; 103(3): 26–32.

99. Girardi, N.L." Blunted Catecholamine Responses after Glucose Ingestion in Children with Attention Deficit Disorder." *Pediatr Res.* 1995; 38: 539–542.

Berdonces, J.L. "Attention Deficit and Infantile Hyperactivity." *Rev Enferm.* Jan 2001; 4(1): 11–4.

100. Lechin, F., et al. "Effects of an Oral Glucose Load on Plasma Neurotransmitters in Humans." *Neuropsychobiology.* 1992; 26(1–2): 4–11.

101. Arieff, A.I. "IVs of Sugar Water Can Cut Off Oxygen to the Brain." Veterans Administration Medical Center in San Francisco. *San Jose Mercury.* Jun 12/86.

102. De Stefani, E. "Dietary Sugar and Lung Cancer: a Case Control Study in Uruguay." *Nutr Cancer.* 1998; 31(2): 132–7.

103. Sandler, B.P. *Diet Prevents Polio.* (Milwakuee, WI: The Lee Foundation for Nutr Research, 1951).

104. Murphy, P. "The Role of Sugar in Epileptic Seizures." *Townsend Letter for Doctors and Patients.* May 2001.

105. Stern, N. and Tuck, M. "Pathogenesis of Hypertension in Diabetes Mellitus." *Diabetes Mellitus, a Fundamental and Clinical Test. 2nd Edition.* (Philadelphia, PA: Lippincott Williams & Wilkins, 2000) 943–957.

Citation Preuss, H.G., et al. "Sugar-Induced Blood Pressure Elevations Over the Lifespan of Three Substrains of Wistar Rats." *J Am Coll Nutr.* 1998; 17(1): 36–37.

106. Christansen, D. "Critical Care: Sugar Limit Saves Lives." *Science News.* Jun 30, 2001; 159: 404.

Donnini, D., et al. "Glucose May Induce Cell Death through a Free Radical-mediated Mechanism." *Biochem Biophys Res Commun.* Feb 15, 1996; 219(2): 412–417.

107. Levine, A.S., et al. "Sugars and Fats: The Neurobiology of Preference " *J Nutr.* 2003; 133: 831S–834S.

108. Schoenthaler, S. "The Los Angeles Probation Department Diet-Behavior Program: Am Empirical Analysis of Six Institutional Settings." *Int J Biosocial Res.* 5(2): 88–89.

109. Deneo-Pellegrini H., et al. "Foods, Nutrients and Prostate Cancer: a Case-control Study in Uruguay." *Br J Cancer.* May 1999; 80(3–4): 591–7.

110. "Gluconeogenesis in Very Low Birth Weight Infants Receiving Total Parenteral Nutrition." *Diabetes.* Apr 1999; 48(4): 791–800.

111. Lenders, C. M. "Gestational Age and Infant Size at Birth Are Associated with Dietary Intake Among Pregnant Adolescents." *J Nutr.* 1998; 128: 807–1810.

112. Peet, M. "International Variations in the Outcome of Schizophrenia and the Prevalence of Depression in Relation to National Dietary Practices: An Ecological Analysis." *Brit J Psy.* 2004; 184: 404–408.

113. Fonseca, V., et al. "Effects of a High-fat-sucrose Diet on Enzymes in Homosysteine Metabolism in the Rat." *Metabolism.* 2000; 49: 736–41.

114. Potischman, N., et al. "Increased Risk of Early-stage Breast Cancer Related to Consumption of Sweet Foods Among Women Less than Age 45 in the United States." *Cancer Causes & Control.* Dec 2002; 13(10): 937–46.

115. Negri, E., et al. "Risk Factors for Adenocarcinoma of the Small Intestine." *Int J Cancer.* Jul 1999; 2(2): 171–4.

116. Bosetti, C., et al. "Food Groups and Laryngeal Cancer Risk: A Case-control Study from Italy and Switzerland." *Int J Cancer.* 2002; 100(3): 355–358.

117. Shannon, M. "An Empathetic Look at Overweight." *CCL Family Found.* Nov-Dec 1993; 20(3): 3–5. POPLINE Document Number: 091975.

118. Harry, G. and Preuss, MD, Georgetown University Medical School. http://www.usa.weekend.com/food/carper_archive/961201carper_eatsmart.html.

119. Beauchamp, G.K., and Moran, M. "Acceptance of Sweet and Salty Tastes in 2-year-old Children." *Appetite.* Dec 1984; 5(4): 291–305.

120. Cleve, T.L. *On the Causation of Varicose Veins.* (Bristol, England: John Wright, 1960).

121. Ket, Yaffe, et al. "Diabetes, Impaired Fasting Glucose and Development of Cognitive Impairment in Older Women." *Neurology.* 2004; 63: 658-663.

122. Chatenoud, Liliane, et al. "Refined-cereal Intake and Risk of Selected Cancers in Italy." *Am J Clin Nutr.* Dec 1999; 70: 1107–1110.

123. Yoo, Sunmi, et al. "Comparison of Dietary Intakes Associated with Metabolic Syndrome Risk Factors in Young Adults: the Bogalusa Heart Study." *Am J Clin Nutr.* Oct 2004; 80(4): 841–848.

124. Shaw, Gary M., et al. "Neural Tube Defects Associated with Maternal Periconceptional Dietary Intake of Simple Sugars and Glycemic Index." *Am J Clin Nutr.* Nov 2003; 78: 972–978.

125. Powers, L. "Sensitivity: You React to What You Eat." *Los Angeles Times.* Feb 12, 1985.

Cheng, J., et al. "Preliminary Clinical Study on the Correlation Between Allergic Rhinitis and Food Factors." *Lin Chuang Er Bi Yan Hou Ke Za Zhi.* Aug 2002; 16(8): 393–396.

126. Jarnerot, G. "Consumption of Refined Sugar by Patients with Crohn's Disease, Ulcerative colitis, or Irritable Bowel Syndrome." *Scand J Gastroenterol.* Nov 1983; 18(8): 999–1002.

127. Allen, S. "Sugars and Fats: The Neurobiology of Preference." *J Nutr.* 2003; 133: 831S-834S.

128. De Stefani, E., et al. "Sucrose as a Risk Factor for Cancer of the Colon and Rectum: a Case-control Study in Uruguay." *Int J Cancer.* Jan 5, 1998; 75(1): 40–4.

129. Levi, F., et al. "Dietary Factors and the Risk of Endometrial Cancer." *Cancer.* Jun 1, 1993; 71(11): 3575–3581.

130. Mellemgaard, A., et al. "Dietary Risk Factors for Renal Cell Carcinoma in Denmark." *Eur J Cancer.* Apr 1996; 32A(4): 673–82.

131. Rogers, A.E., et al. "Nutritional and Dietary Influences on Liver Tumorigenesis in Mice and Rats." *Arch Toxicol Suppl.* 1987; 10: 231–43. Review.

132. Sørensen, L.B., et al. "Effect of Sucrose on Inflammatory Markers in Overweight Humans" *Am J Clin Nutr.* Aug 2005; 82(2).

133. Smith, R.N., et al. "The Effect of a High-protein, Low Glycemic-load Diet Versus a Conventional, High Glycemic-load Diet on Biochemical Parameters Associated with Acne Vulgaris: A Randomized, Investigator-masked, Controlled Trial." *J Am Acad Dermatol.* 2007; 57: 247–256.

134. Selva, D.M., et al. "Monosaccharide-induced Lipogenesis Regulates the Human Hepatic Sex Hormone-binding Globulin Gene." *J Clin Invest.* 2007. doi:10.1172/JCI32249.

135. Krietsch, K., et al. "Prevalence, Presenting Symptoms, and Psychological Characteristics of Individuals Experiencing a Diet-related Mood-disturbance." *Behavior Therapy.* 1988; 19(4): 593–604.

136. Berglund, M., et al. "Comparison of Monounsaturated Fat with Carbohydrates as a Replacement for Saturated Fat in Subjects with a High Metabolic Risk Profile: Studies in the Fasting and Postprandial States." *Am J Clin Nutr.* Dec 1, 2007; 86(6): 1611–1620.

137. Gao, X., et al. "Intake of Added Sugar and Sugar-Sweetened Drink and Serum Uric Acid Concentration in US Men and Women." *Hypertension.* Aug 1, 2007; 50(2): 306–312.

138. Wu, T., et al. Fructose, Glycemic Load, and Quantity and Quality of Carbohydrate in Relation to Plasma C-peptide Concentrations in US Women." *Am J Clin Nutr.* Oct 2004; (4):1043–1049.

139. Matthias, B. and Schulze, M.B. "Dietary Pattern, Inflammation, and Incidence of Type 2 Diabetes in Women." *Am J Clin Nutr.* Sep 2005; 82: 675–684.

140. Yudkin, J. *Sweet and Dangerous.* (New York: Bantam Books: 1974) 169.

Chapter 3

1. Eck, P. Analytical Research Labs, Inc., 2338.

2. Albrecht, W. "The Albrecht Papers." www.earthmentor.comprinciples_of_balance/doctor_albrecht_papers/.

3. Ashmead, D. *Chelated Mineral Nutrition.* International Institute of Natural Health Sciences, Inc. 1979.

4. Paganelli, R., et al. "Detection of Specific Antigen Within Circulating Immune Complexes: Validation of the Assay and its Application to Food Antigen-Antibody Complexes Formed in Healthy and Food-Allergic Subjects." *Clin Exp Immunol.* Oct 1981; 46(1): 44–53.

5. Warshaw, A.L., et al. "Protein Uptake by the Intestine: Evidence for Absorption of Intact Macromolecules." *Gastroenter.* 1974; 66: 987.

6. Philpott, W. *Brain Allergies.* (New Canaan, CT: Keats Publishing, Inc. 1980).

7. Paganelli, R., et al. "The Role of Antigenic Absorption and Circulating Immune Complexes in Food Allergy." *Ann Allergy.* 1986; 57: 330–336.

8. Taylor, B., et al. "Transient IgA Deficiency and Pathogenesis of Infantile Atopy." *Lancet.* 1973; 2: 11.

9. Stevens, W.J., and Bridts, C.H. "IgG-containing and IgE-containing Circulating Immune Complexes in Patients with Asthma and Rhinitis." *J All Clin Immun.* 1979; 63: 297.

10. Hyatum, M., et al. "The Gut-Joint Axis: Cross Reactive Food Antibodies in Rheumatoid Arthritis." *Gut.* Sep 2006; 55(9): 1240–1247.

11. Catteral, W.E., et al. "Placebo-Controlled, Blind Study of Dietary Manipulation Therapy in Rheumatoid Arthritis." *Lancet.* Feb 6, 1986; 236–238.

12. Jones, H.D. "Management of Multiple Sclerosis." *Postgrad Med J.* May 1952; 2: 415–422.

13. Douglas, J.M. "Psoriasis and Diet." *West J Med.* Nov 1980; 133: 450.

14. Brostoff, J., et al. "Production of IgE Complexes by Allergen Challenge in Atopic Patients and the Effect of Sodium Cromoglycate." *Lancet.* 1979; 1: 1267.

15. Jackson, P.G., et al. "Intestinal Permeability in Patients with Eczema and Food Allergy." *Lancet.* 1981; 1: 1285.

16. Wright, R. and Truelove, S.C. "Circulating Antibodies to Dietary Proteins in Ulcerative Colitis." *Brit Med J.* 1965; 2: 142.

17. Penn, A.H., et al. "Pancreatic Enzymes Generate Cytotoxic Mediators in the Intestine." *Shock.* Mar 2007; 27(3): 296–304.

18. Kijak, E., et al. "Relationship of Blood Sugar Level and Leukocytic Phagocytosis." *J South California Dental Assoc.* Sep 1964; 32: 9.

19. Sanchez, A., et al. "Role of Sugars in Human Neutrophilic Phagocytosis." *Amer J Epidemiol.* 1992; 135(8): 895–903.

20. Selye, H. *The Stress of Life*. (San Francisco: McGraw-Hill, 1978).

21. Editorial. "Depression, Stress and Immunity." *Lancet*. 1987; 1: 1467–1468.

Chapter 4

1. Madden, K.M., et al. "The Oral Glucose Tolerance Test Induces Mycardial Ischemia in Healthy Older Adults." *Clin Invest Med*. 2007; 30(3): E118–E126.

2. Ko, G.T., et al. "The Reproducibility and Usefulness of the Oral Glucose Tolerance Test in Screening for Diabetes and Other Cardiovascular Risk Factors." *Ann Clin Biochem*. Jan 1998; 35(Pt 1): 62–67.

3. Philpott, W.H. and Kalita, D.K. *Victory Over Diabetes*. (New York: McGraw-Hill, 1991).

4. Fan, L.F. "Study of Causes of Untoward Reactions of the Glucose Tolerance Test." *Zhonghua Hu Li Za Zhi*. Jul 5, 1994; 29(7): 387–390.

5. Geberhiwot, T., et al. "HbA1c Predicts the Likelihood of Having Impaired Glucose Tolerance in High-risk Patients with Normal Fasting Plasma Glucose." *Ann Clin Biochem*. May 2005; 42(Pt 3): 193–195.

6. Peters, H.L., et al. "To Determine Whether a Glycosylated Hemoglobin Level Can Be Used in Place of an Oral Glucose Tolerance Test (OGTT) to Diagnose Diabetes." *JAMA*. Oct 16, 1999; 276(15): 1246–1252.

7. Novak, B.J. "Exhaled Methyl Nitrate as a Noninvasive Marker of Hyperglycemia in Type 1 Diabetes." *Proceed of Nat Acad Science*. Oct 2, 2007; 104(40): 15613–15618.

Chapter 5

1. U.S. Department of Agriculture. "Food Availability: Custom Queries." www.ers.usda.gov/Data/FoodConsumption/FoodAvailQueriable.aspx.

2. Ibid.

3. Ibid.

4. Taras, H.L., et al. "Policy Statement." *Pediatrics*. Jan 2004; 113; 1: 152–154.

5. Ludwig, D.S., et al. "Relation Between Consumption of Sugar-Sweetened Drinks and Childhood Obesity: a Prospective Observational Analysis." *Lancet*. 2001; 57: 505–508.

6. Mattes, R.D. "Dietary Compensation in Humans for Supplemental Energy Provided as Ethanol or Carbohydrates in Fluids." *Physiol Behav*. 1999; 99: 436–441.

7. "Why Soda is Bad for You." www.mercola.com. Viewed Dec 21, 2007.

8. Tordoff, M.G. and Alleva, A.M. "Effect of Drinking Soda Sweetened with Aspartame or High Fructose Corn Syrup on Food Intake and Body Weight." *Am J Clin Nutr*. 1990; 51: 963–969.

9. Peppa, M., et al. "Glucose, Advanced Glycation End Products, and Diabetes Complications: What Is New and What Works." *Clin Diabetes*. 2003; 21: 186–187.

10. USDA. "Food Consumption." http://ers.usda.gov/publications/sb965/sb965f.pdf. Projected upon 1997's consumption. Page 9.

11. Uribarri, J., et al. "Diet-Derived Advanced Glycation End Products Are Major Contributors to the Body's AGE Pool and Induce Inflammation in Healthy Subjects." *Annals N Y Acad Sci*. 2005: 461–466.

12. Tabaton, M., et al. "Is Amyloid Beta-protein Glycated in Alzheimer's Disease?" *Neuroreport*. 1997; 8(4): 907–909.

13. Ishibashi, T., et al. "Advanced Glycation End Products in Age-related Macular Degeneration."*Arch Ophthalmol*. Dec 1998; 116(12): 1629–1632.

14. Dawczynski, E. "Advanced Glycation End-Products (AGEs) and Cataract—Distribution in Different Types of Cataract." www.dog.org/2001/abstract_german/Dawczynski_e.htm. Viewed Oct 22, 2007.

15. Drinda, S. "Identification of the Advanced Glycation End Products N (epsilon)-carboxymethyllysine in the Synovial Tissue of Patients with Rheumatoid Arthritis."*Ann Rheum Dis*. Jun 2002; 61(6): 488–492.

16. Vlassara, H. Picower Institute for Medical Research in Manhasset, N.Y.; Annual meeting of the American Diabetes Association in San Francisco. Jun 1996.

17. Krajcovicova-Kudlackova, M., et al. "Advanced Glycation End Products and Nutrition." *Physiol Res*. 2002; 51: 313–316.

18. Peppa, M., et al. "Glucose, Advanced Glycation End Products, and Diabetes Complications: What Is New and What Works." *Clin Diabetes*. 2003; 21: 186–187.

19. King, R.H.M. "The Role of Glycation in the Pathogenesis of Diabetic Polyneuropathy." *J Clin Pathol: Mol Pathol*. 2001; 54: 400–408.

20. Bunn, F., and Higgins, P.J. "Reaction of Monosaccharides with Protein: Possible Evolutionary Significance." *Science*. Jul 10, 1981: 213.

21. Nutrient Data Laboratory, Beltsville Human Nutrition Research Center (BHNRC), Agricultural Research Service (ARS), U.S. Department of Agriculture (USDA). "USDA Database for the Added Sugars Content of Selected Foods." www.nal.usda.gov/fnic/foodcomp/Data/add_sug/addsug01.pdf.

22. USDA Agricultural Research Service. "USDA Database for the Added Sugars Content of Selected Foods, Release 1." www.ars.usda.gov/Services/docs.htm?docid=12107.

23. National Diabetes Clearing House. "Total Prevalence of Diabetes in the United States, All Ages, 2005." http://diabetes.niddk.nih.gov/dm/pubs/statistics/index.htm.

24. Hallfrisch, J. "Metabolic Effects of Dietary Fructose." *FASEB J*. Jun 1990; 4: 2652–2660.

25. Bunn, H.F. and Higgins, P.J. "Reaction of Monosaccharides with Proteins; Possible Evolutionary Significance." *Science.* 1981; 213: 2222–2244.

26. Dills, W.L. "Protein Fructosylation: Fructose and the Maillard Reaction." *Am J Clin Nutr.* 1993; 58(suppl): 779S–787S.

27. Hallfrisch, J., et al. "The Effects of Fructose on Blood Lipid Levels." *Am J Clin Nutr.* 1983; 37(3): 740–748.

28. Hollenbeck, C.B. "Dietary Fructose Effects on Lipoprotein Metabolism and Risk for Coronary Artery Disease." *Am J Clin Nutr.* 1993; 58(suppl): 800S–807S.

29. Bantle, J.P. "Effects of Dietary Fructose on Plasma Lipids in Healthy Subjects." *Am J Clin Nutr.* Nov 2000; 72: 1128–1134.

30. Rumessen, J.J. and Gudmand-Hoyer, E. "Functional Bowel Disease: Malabsorption and Abdominal Distress After Ingestion of Fructose, Sorbitol, and Fructose-Sorbitol Mixtures." *Gastroenterol.* Sep 1988; 95(3): 694–700.

31. Ledochowski, M., et al. "Fructose Malabsorption is Associated with Early Signs of Mental Depression." *Eur J Med Res.* Jun 17, 1998; 3(6): 295–298.

32. Macdonald, J., et al. "Some Effects, in Man, of Varying the Load of Glucose, Sucrose, Fructose, or Sorbitol on Various Metabolites in Blood." *Am J Clin Nutr.* Aug 1978; 31: 1305–1311.

33. Hallfrisch, J., et al. "The Effects of Fructose on Blood Lipid Levels." *Am J Clin Nutr.* 1983; 37(3): 740–748.

34. Bender, A.E. and Damji, K.B. "Some Effects of Dietary Sucrose." *World Review of Nutrition and Dietetics.* 1972; 15: 104–155.

35. Zakim, D. and Herman, R.H. "Fructose Metabolism II." *Am J Clin Nutr.* 1968; 21: 315–319.

36. Hunter, B.T. "Confusing Consumers About Sugar Intake." *Consumer's Research.* Jan 1995; 78(1): 14–17.

37. McDonald, R.B. "Influence of Dietary Sucrose on Biological Aging." *Am J Clin Nutr.* 1995; 62(suppl): 284S–293S.

38. Bergstra, A.E., et al. "Dietary Fructose vs. Glucose Stimulates Nepphrocalcinogensis in Female Rats." *J Nutr.* Jul 1993; 123(7): 1320–1327.

39. Ivaturi, R. and Kies, C. "Mineral Balances in Humans as Affected by Fructose, High Fructose Corn Syrup and Sucrose." *Plant Foods for Human Nutrition.* 1992; 42(2): 143–151.

40. Fields, M. "The Severity of Copper Deficiency in Rats is Determined by the Type of Dietary Carbohydrate." *Proceedings of the Society of Experimental Biology and Medicine.* 1984; 175: 530–537.

41. Teff, K.L., et al. "Dietary Fructose Reduces Circulating Insulin and Leptin, Attenuates Postprandial Suppression of Ghrelin, and Increases Triglycerides in Women." *J Clin Endocrin Metab.* Jun 4, 2004; 89(6): 2963–2972.

42. Bayard, V., et al. "Does Flavanol Intake Influence Mortality from Nitric Oxide-Dependent Processes? Ischemic Heart Disease, Stroke, Diabetes Mellitus and Cancer in Panama." *Int J Med Sci.* 2007; 4: 53–58.

43. Gu, L., et al. "Procyanidin and Catechin Contents and Antioxidant Capacity of Cocoa and Chocolate Products." *J Agric Food Chem.* May 31, 2006; 54(11): 4057–4061.

44. The History of Chocolate. "Chocolate Necessities." www.chocolatenecessities.com/history_of_chocolate.php.

45. Gee, J.M., et al. "Effects of Conventional Sucrose-Based, Fructose-Based and Isomalt-Based Chocolates on Postprandial Metabolism in Non-Insulin Dependent Diabetics." *Eur J Clin Nutr.* Nov 1991; 45(11): 561–566.

46. Mars, Incorporated. "CocoaVia Snacks Nutrition Facts." www.cocoavia.com/products/nutrition_facts.aspx.

47. Center for Science in the Public Interest. "Food Additives." http://cspinet.org/reports/chemcuisine.htm.

48. Tomaso, E., et al. "Brain Cannabinoids in Chocolate." *Nature.* 1996; 382: 677–678.

49. Cambria, S., et al. "Hyperexcitability Syndrome in a Newborn Infant of Chocoholic Mother." *Am J Perinatol.* Oct 2006; 23(7): 421–422.

50. Hodgson, J.M., et al. "Chocolate Consumption and Bone Density in Older Women." *Am J Clin Nutr.* Jan 2008; 87(1): 175–180.

Chapter 6

1. Flegal, K.M., et al. "Prevalence and Trends in Obesity Among US Adults, 1999–2002." *JAMA.* 2002; 288: 1723–1727.

2. Shankuan, Z., et al. "Waist Circumference and Obesity-associated Risk Factors among Whites in the Third National Health and Nutrition Examination Survey: Clinical Action Thresholds." *Am J Clin Nutr.* Oct 2002; 76(4): 743.

3. Tannous, et al. "Variations in Postprandial Ghrelin Status Following Ingestion of High-Carbohydrate, High-Fat and High-Protein Meals in Males." *Ann Nutr Metab.* Feb 2006; 50(3): 260–269.

4. U.S. Census Bureau. "Statisical Abstract of the United States, 2002, Table 195." www.census.gov/prod/2003pubs/02statab/health.pdf.

5. Elliot, S., et al. "Fructose, Weight Gain and the Insulin Resistance Syndrome." *Am J Clin Nutr.* Nov 2002; 76(53): 911–922.

6. "Is Fructose Bad For You?" *Harvard Health Letter.* May 1, 2007.

7. Bingham, S., et al. "Epidemiologic Assessment of Sugars Consumption Using Biomarkers: Comparisons of Obese and Non-obese Individuals." *Cancer Epidemiol Biomarkers Prev.* 2007; 16: 1651–1654.

8. Avena, N.M., et al. "Evidence for sugar addiction: behavioral and neurochem-

ical effects of intermittent, excessive sugar intake." *Neuroscience & Biobehavioral Reviews.* 2008; 32(1): 20–39.

9. Stephanie, et al. "A Maternal 'Junk Food' Diet in Pregnancy and Lactation Promotes an Exacerbated Taste for 'Junk Food' and a Greater Propensity for Obesity in Rat Offspring." *Brit J Nutr.* Oct 2007; 98(4): 843–851.

10. Turnbaugh, P.T., et al. "An Obesity-Associated Gut Microbiome with Increased Capacity for Energy Harvest." *Nature.* Feb 2002; 444: 21.

11. Ley, R.E., et al. "Microbial Ecology: Human Gut Microbes Associated with Obesity." *Nature.* Dec 21, 2006; 444: 21–28.

12. Center for Disease Control. "Overweight and Obesity." www.jhsph.edu/pub- lichealthnews/press_releases/2007/wang_adult_obesity.html. Viewed Dec 12, 2008.

13. Segal, M.S., et al. "Is the Fructose Index More Relevant with Regards to Cardiovascular Disease than the Glycemic Index?" *Eur J Nutr.* Oct 2007; 46(7): 406–417.

14. Young, L.R. and Nestle, M. "Expanding Portion Sizes in the US Marketplace: Implications for Nutrition Counseling." *Journal of the American Dietetic Association.* 103(2): 231–234L .

15. Allison, et al. "Annual Deaths Attributable to Obesity in the U.S." *JAMA.* Oct 1999; 282: 1530–1538.

16. Glinsman, W., et al. "Report from FDA's Sugars Task Force, 1986: Evaluation of Health Aspects of Sugars Contained in Carbohydrate Sweeteners." Food and Drug Administration. 1986: 42.

17. Crook, W. "Why Does the Ingestion of Sugar Cause Hyperactivity in Many Children?" *Townsend Letter for Doctors.* Jul 1992: 581–582.

18. School Library Journal Staff."Kids Less Likely to Graduate High School Than Parents." *School Library J.* Oct 27, 2008.

19. "18 Big Ideas to Fix the Health Care System." *Reader's Digest.* www.rd.com/ living-healthy/18-ideas-to-reform-health-care-now/article101364–1.html; www.Healthykidshelathycommunities.org; www.healthykidssmartkids.com.

20. Lien, L. "Consumption of Soft Drinks and Hyperactivity, Mental Distress, and Conduct Problems Among Adolescents in Oslo, Norway." *Am J Public Health.* Oct 2006; 96(101): 1815–1820.

21. Keller, K.B, and Lemberg, L. "Obesity and the Metabolic Syndrome." *Am J Crit Care.* 2003; 12: 167–170.

22. American Heart Association. "Metabolic Syndrome." www.americanheart. org/presenter.jhtml?identifier=4756.

23. Shankuan, Z., et. al. "Waist Circumference and Obesity-associated Risk Factors among Whites in the Third National Health and Nutrition Examination Survey: Clinical Action Thresholds." *Am J Clin Nutr.* Oct 2002; 76(4): 743.

24. Sang, W.O., et al. "Association Between Cigarette Smoking and Metabolic Syndrome." *Diabetes Care.* 2005; 28: 2064–2066.

25. Rett, K. "The Relation between Insulin Resistance and Cardiovascular Complications of the Insulin Resistance Syndrome." *Diabetes Obes Metab.* 1999; 1(Sup.1): S8–S16.

26. Astrup, A. and Finer, N. "Redefining Type-2 Diabetes: 'Diabesity' or 'Obesity Dependent Diabetes Mellitus'?" *Obes Rev.* 2000; 1: 57–59.

27. Mokdad, A.H., et al. "Diabetes Trends in the US: 1990–1998." *Diabetes Care.* 2000; 23: 1278–1283.

28. Pan, X.R., et al. "Prevalence of Diabetes and its Risk Factors in China, 1994, National Diabetes Prevention and Control Cooperative Group." *Diabetes Care.* 1997; 20: 1664–1669.

29. Ramachandran, A., et al. "Rising Prevalence of NIDDM in an Urban Population in India." *Diabetologia.* 1997; 40: 232–237.

30. Centers for Disease Control and Prevention NCIHS, Division of Health Interview Statistics: Census of the Population and Population Estimates. (Hyattsville, MD: Centers for Disease Control and Prevention, 1997).

31. Zimmet, P., et al. "Global and Societal Implications of the Diabetes Epidemic." *Nature.* 2001; 414: 782–787.

32. Freedman, D.S., et al. "Relationship of Childhood Obesity to Coronary Heart Disease Risk Factors in Adulthood: the Bogalusa Heart Study." *Pediatrics.* 2001; 108: 712–718.

33. Yaffe, K., et al. "The Metabolic Syndrome, Inflammation, and Risk of Cognitive Decline." *JAMA.* Nov 10, 2004; 292(18): 2237–2242.

34. Merz, C.N., et al. "Effects of a Randomized Controlled Trial of Transcendental Meditation on Components of the Metabolic Syndrome in Subjects with Coronary Heart Disease." *Arch Intern Med.* 2006; 166(11): 1218–1224.

35. Kromhout, D., et al. "Dietary Saturated and Trans Fatty Acids and Cholesterol and 25-year Mortality From Coronary Heart Disease: the Seven Countries Study." *Prev Med.* 1995; 24: 308–315.

36. Liu, S. and Manson, J.E. "Dietary Carbohydrates, Physical Inactivity, Obesity and the 'Metabolic Syndrome' as Predictors of Coronary Heart Disease." *Curr Opin Lipidol.* 2001; 12: 395–404.

37. Dhingra, R., et al. "Soft drink Consumption and Risk of Developing Cardiometabolic Risk factors and the Metabolic Syndrome in Middle-aged Adults in the Community." *Circulation.* Jul 31, 2007; 116(5): 480–488.

38. Esposito, K., et al. "Effect of a Mediterranean-Style Diet on Endothelial Dysfunction and Markers of Vascular Inflammation in the Metabolic Syndrome: a Randomized Trial." *JAMA.* Sep 22/29, 2004; 292(12): 1440–1446.

39. Esmaillzade, A. "Fruit and Vegetable Intakes, C-reactive protein, and the Metabolic Syndrome." *Am J Clin Nutr.* Dec 2006; 84(6): 1489–1497.

40. Yaffe, K., et al. "Diabetes, Impaired Fasting Glucose and Development of Cognitive Impairment in Older Women." *Neurology.* 2004; 63: 658–663.

41. Whitmer, R.A., et al. "Obesity in Middle Age and Future Risk of Dementia: a 27–Year Longitudinal Population Based Study." *Brit Med J.* Jun 11, 2005; 330(7504): 1360.

42. Okereke, O., et al. "Plasma C Peptide Level and Cognitive Function Among Women Without Diabetes Mellitus." *Arch Intern Med.* Jul 25, 2005; 165(14): 1651–1656.

43. Munshi, M., et al. "Cognitive Dysfunction Is Associated With Poor Diabetes Control in Older Adults." *Diabetes Care.* Aug 1, 2006; 29(8): 1794–1799.

44. American Cancer Society. "What is Cancer?" www.cancer.org/docroot/CRI/content/CRI_2_4_1x_What_Is_Cancer.asp?sitearea=.

45. Warburg, O. "The Chemical Constitution of Respiration Ferment." *Science.* Nov 9, 1928; 68(1767): 437–443.

46. Radiology Info. www.radiologyinfo.org/en/info.cfm?pg=PET&bhcp=1.

47. Children's Hospital of Boston. www.childrenshospital.org/az/Site2154/mainpageS2154P0.html.

48. Michaud, D.S., et al. "Dietary Sugar, Glycemic Load and Pancreatic Cancer Risk in a Prospective Study." *National Cancer Institute.* Sep 4, 2000; 94(17): 1293–1300.

49. Danhauer, S.C., et al. "A Survey of Cancer Patient Preferences: Which types of Snacks Do They Prefer during Treatment?" *European Journal of Cancer Care.* Jan 2009; 18(1): 37–42.

50. Michels, K.B., et al. "Type-2 Diabetes and Subsequent Incidence of Breast Cancer in the Nurse's Health Study." *Diabetes Care.* Jun 2003; 26(6): 1752–1758.

51. De Stefani, E., et al. "Dietary Sugar and Lung Cancer: a Case-Control Study in Uruguay." *Nutr Cancer.* 1998; 31(2): 132–137.

52. De Stefani, E., et al. "Sucrose as a Risk Factor for Cancer of the Colon and Rectum: a Case-Control Study in Uruguay." *Int J Cancer.* Jan 5, 1998; 75(1): 40–44.

53. Santisteban, G.A., et al. "Glycemic Modulation of Tumor Tolerance in a Mouse Model of Breast Cancer." *Biochem Biophys Res Commun.* Nov 15, 1995; 132(3): 1174–1179.

54. McClintock, M.K., et al. "Cancer risks associated with Life Events and Conflict Solution." *J Gerontol B Psychol Sci Soc Sci.* Mar 2005; 60(Spec No 1): 32–41.

55. Galic, M.A. and Persinger, M.A. "Sucrose Ingestion Decreases Seizure Onset Time in Female Rats Treated with Lithium and Pilocarpine." *Epilepsy & Behavior.* Jun 2005; 6(4): 552–555.

56. The Epilepsy Foundation. "The Ketogenic Diet." www.epilepsyfoundation. org/about/treatment/ketogenicdiet/ketoteam.cfm.

Chapter 7

1. Catlin, et al. "National Health Spending in 2005." *Health Affairs*. 2006; 26(1): 142–153.

2. Borger, C., et al. "Health Spending Projections Through 2015: Changes on the Horizon." *Health Affairs Web Exclusive*. W61.

3. The National Coalition on Health Care. "Health Insurance Costs." www.nchc.org/ facts/cost.shtml.

4. Pear, R. "U.S. Health Care Spending Reaches All-Time High: 15% of GDP." *The New York Times*. Jan 9, 2004: 3.

5. U.S. Census Bureau, International Database. Shown on Website: Infoplease.* www.infoplease.com/pa/A0934746.html.

6. U.S. Census Bureau, International Database. Shown on Website: Infoplease.* www.infoplease.com/pa/A0934744.html.

7. World Health Organization. Shown on Website: Infoplease.* www.infoplease. com/world/statistics/obesity.html.

8. Edwaurd, C. "Why Congress Should Appeal the Sugar Subsidy." The Cato Institute. www.cato.org/pub_display.php?pub_id=8381.

About the Authors

Nancy Appleton earned her BS in clinical nutrition from UCLA and her PhD in health services from Walden University. She graduated with honors from Walden University with her award-winning dissertation, *An Alternative to the Germ Theory*. She has retired from her private practice and lives in San Diego, but continues to research, lecture, and write about nutrition and health issues. She appears regularly on radio, TV, and Internet broadcasts. In addition to *Suicide by Sugar*, she has written several books on nutrition and health: *Stopping Inflammation*, *Healthy Bones*, *Lick the Sugar Habit*, *Lick the Sugar Habit Sugar Counter*, and *Curse of Louis Pasteur*.

G.N. Jacobs (Greg to his friends) is a reporter, novelist, essayist, and many other job titles that involve words on paper. He is proud of his first novel *Blood & Ink* and his subsequent short story collection, *The Beast that Almost Ate Los Angeles*. His work with Dr. Appleton started out as a client and blossomed from there. He also co-wrote *Stopping Inflammation* with Dr. Appleton. He lives in Los Angeles where he writes several blogs, including one about Star Trek. Presently, he's hard at work on several new books.

Index

Abbott Laboratories, 47, 50
Addiction, sugar
    definition of, 6
    how to tell if you have a, 9
    studies on, by Magalie Lenoir,
        8–9
    studies on, by Nicole Avena, 8
    ways to break a, 109–110
Advanced Glycated End Products
    (AGEs)
    diseases and, 54–55
    relationship to sugar, 53–54
    ways to slow progression of,
        55–56
Alzheimer's disease. *See* Dementia.
American Academy of Pediatrics
    (AAP), 42
American Diabetes Association, 54
American Journal of Perinatology, 69
American Medical Association
    (AMA), 92
Anandamide, 68. *See also* Choco-
    late, reasons besides
        sugar not to eat.
Avena, Nicole. *See* Addiction,
    sugar, studies on by Nicole
        Avena.

Bacteroidetes. *See* Obesity, studies
    on, by Jeffrey Gordon; Obesity,
    studies on, by Marie Collado.
Baked beets, recipe for, 122–123. *See
    also* Recipes.
Beech-Nut, 52
Beet root dessert, recipe for, 125. *See
    also* Recipes.
Beltsville Human Nutrition
        Research Center's Community
        Nutrition Research Group, 57
Body mass index (BMI), calculation
    for, 44
Body Monitor Kit, 82, 111
Brain Allergies (Philpott), 24
Breathalyzer-style glucose test. *See*
    Oral glucose tolerance test
    (OGTT), options to consider
    before taking.
Buono, Victor, 77–78

Caffeine in chocolate, 67–68. *See
    also* Chocolate, reasons besides
        sugar not to eat.
Calcium-phosphorus ratio, 45
Cancer, 96
    causes of, 96–97

Order Forms

AUDIO CDS

Lick the Sugar Habit—An introduction to the book of the same name, this disk provides detailed explanations of the body chemistry principle, mineral relationships, enzyme function, and causes of infectious and degenerative disease. (1 hour)

Allergies—What are food allergies? What causes them? How can they be eliminated? Learn how foods to which you have allergic reactions can be reintroduced to your diet. The similar role of environmental allergies is also discussed. (1 hour)

Osteoporosis—Although you may be getting enough calcium in your diet, if you're out of homeostasis, this mineral can't be absorbed properly. This disk explains how to look for symptoms of calcium deficiency and how to test for susceptibility to osteoporosis. (1 hour)

Women/Obesity—A combined disk with two sections starting with the latest information concerning pre-menstrual syndrome, Candida (yeast) infections, menstruation, menopause, and post-menopause problems. The second section relates information about the latest research on the relationship of allergies, addictions, and cravings to obesity. (1 hour)

Children—This disk begins with prenatal nutrition and continues with information about food allergies and eating problems in children. Ideas for convincing children of all ages to eat nutritious foods fill out the end of the tape. (1 hour)

Food Preparation—This disk answers some important questions. Where can I shop for the most nutritious foods? How should I prepare food to preserve health and maintain my and my family's body chemistry? What about additives, irradiation, pesticides, and fungicides? (1 hour)

The Body Monitor—How do you test for homeostasis with urine and saliva testing? What are the common causes for being out of homeostasis? How do you regain homeostasis once you are out? This disk answers these questions. (45 minutes)

Diet and the Immune System—This disk presents an overview of the whole Body Chemistry Principle in this recording made live in 1996. Dr. Appleton explains many things and answers questions from the audience. (78 minutes)

Additional Information—Dr. Appleton naturally found more information to present after recording the disks above. This CD covers a wide variety of topics left unsaid on other recordings. (1 hour)

AUDIO CDS ORDER FORM

Name:_____

Address: _____ Apt._____

City: _____

State: _____ Zip: _____

List CD Titles:

1. _____   6. _____

2. _____   7. _____

3. _____   8. _____

4. _____   9. _____

5. _____

Price List (U.S. Currency)

Quantity	Price	Shipping
1 CD	$8.00	$2.50
Additional CDs	$8.00 each	$.50 each
All 9 CDs	$50.00	$6.00

California residents must include local sales tax or 9.75%.

Foreign Orders: Canadian residents may use this form, but residents of other countries are requested to use our online ordering system at www.nancy appleton.com to shorten response time and properly deal with the varying postage costs for foreign countries. Canadian residents must send an International Money Order in U.S. Funds, as personal checks may not clear.

To order: Please send a check or money order made out to
Nancy Appleton, PhD with a copy of this form to:
Nancy Appleton Books
5950 Buckingham Parkway
Culver City, CA 90230

You can also contact Nancy Appleton at
nancyappletonbooks@yahoo.com
or visit her website at www.nancyappleton.com.

BODY MONITOR TEST KIT

This kit contains testing materials to determine if your body is in homeostasis, or balance. Included are a bottle of solution for 250 urine tests, two test tubes, pipe cleaner, an eyedropper, a roll of pH paper, and the 28-page instruction booklet *How to Monitor Your Basic Health*. The instructions explain how to test your urine for calcium and properly read the results. The instructions also include information on using the pH paper to test the acidity/alkalinity of both urine and saliva. Information on how to relate these results to your health, along with suggestions for the many things you can do to improve your health, are also presented—especially how the kit may be used to test for allergies. Nancy Appleton Books also adds, at no extra charge, two audio CDs: "Body Monitor" and "Diet and the Immune System" in order to provide additional understanding of the Body Chemistry Principle.

Name:_____

Address: _____ Apt._____

City: _____

State: _____ Zip: _____

Price List (U.S. Currency)

Quantity	Price	Shipping
1 Kit	$33.00	$8.00

California residents must include local sales tax or 9.75%.

Foreign Orders: Canadian residents may use this form, but residents of other countries are requested to use our online ordering system at www.nancyappleton.com to shorten response time and properly deal with the varying postage costs for foreign countries. Canadian residents must send an International Money Order in U.S. Funds, as personal checks may not clear.

To order: Please send a check or money order made out to
Nancy Appleton, PhD with a copy of this form to:
Nancy Appleton Books
5950 Buckingham Parkway
Culver City, CA 90230

You can also contact Nancy Appleton at
nancyappletonbooks@yahoo.com
or visit her website at www.nancyappleton.com.

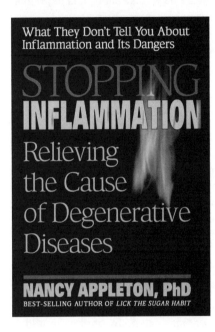

What They Don't Tell You About
Inflammation and Its Dangers

STOPPING
INFLAMMATION

Relieving
the Cause
of Degenerative
Diseases

NANCY APPLETON, PhD
BEST-SELLING AUTHOR OF *LICK THE SUGAR HABIT*

STOPPING INFLAMMATION
Relieving the Cause of Degenerative Diseases
Nancy Appleton, PhD

Most of us think of inflammation as a symptom associated with an infection or injury. Dr. Nancy Appleton, however, has discovered that it might be more than just a simple reaction to a health disorder. When the body's tissues are disturbed in some manner, a series of complex reactions takes place, resulting in inflammation. In most cases, when the disorder stops, the tissue returns to its normal healthy state. Sometimes, though, the tissue remains chronically inflamed. Dr. Appleton's research demonstrates that this condition might be more harmful than ever suspected.

Drawing on the latest medical research, *Stopping Inflammation* begins with a full explanation of inflammation and its causes. It then looks at inflammation's role in various health disorders, from obesity to cancer. Finally, the book provides a number of nondrug treatments aimed not at controlling the problem, but at removing its cause. Here are safe and credible solutions for restoring good health.

$14.95 • 224 pages • 6 x 9-inch quality paperback • Health • ISBN 978-0-7570-0418-2

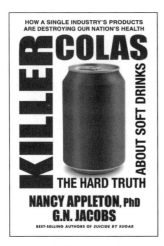

KILLER COLAS
The Hard Truth About Soft Drinks
Nancy Appleton, PhD, and G.N. Jacobs

It's as American as fast food, ice cream, and apple pie. So why are people saying all those nasty things about soda? The answer is simple: Those nasty things are all true. While the facts may be hard to swallow, it is high time we address the damage being done to our well-being due to our long-running love affair with soft drinks and other sweetened beverages. In *Killer Colas,* Dr. Nancy Appleton and G.N. Jacobs provide a startling picture of an industry hell-bent on making a hefty profit at the ultimate expense of the country's health.

Over the last few decades, the sale of soft drinks, energy beverages, sports drinks, and enhanced waters has exploded, as has the incidence of obesity, diabetes, hypertension, heart disease, cancer, and stroke. *Killer Colas* looks at the origin of this downward spiral. The book traces the history and staggering growth of the soft drink industry, explores the powerful influence it has achieved through media-savvy advertising and marketing techniques, and examines the many harmful ingredients that these companies include in their most prized and popular formulas. In addition, it offers evidence of the frighteningly addictive properties of soft drinks, as well as research that links America's consumption of sweetened beverages to its overall decline in health.

In light of the country's overwhelming health crisis, the consequences of drinking soda and other sweetened beverages can no longer be ignored. *Killer Colas* exposes the facts behind a habit that is just as dangerous and destructive as smoking. Moreover, it suggests concrete solutions to this widespread problem, giving hope to a nation desperately in need of a healthful way forward. Once you have read this book, you will never look at soft drinks in the same way again.

Nancy Appleton, PhD, earned her BS in clinical nutrition from UCLA and her PhD in health services from Walden University. She maintains a private practice in Santa Monica, California. An avid researcher, Dr. Appleton lectures extensively throughout the world and has appeared on numerous television and radio talk shows. She is the best-selling author of *Stopping Inflammation, Suicide by Sugar,* and *Healthy Bones.*

G.N. Jacobs is a general reporter and a filmmaker with features, shorts, and documentaries to his credit. Mr. Jacobs runs the online literary magazine *Smoking Lizard.* He currently lives in Los Angeles, California.

$15.95 • 204 pages • 6 x 9-inch paperback • Health • ISBN 978-0-7570-0257-1